W9-DEA-717

DEADLY DISEASES AND EPIDEMICS

MENINGITIS

Anthrax

Campylobacteriosis

Cholera

Escherichia coli Infections

Gonorrhea

Hepatitis

Herpes

HIV/AIDS

Influenza

Lyme Disease

Mad Cow Disease (Bovine Spongiform Encephalopathy)

Malaria

Meningitis

Mononucleosis

Plague

Polio

SARS

Smallpox

Streptococcus (Group A)

Syphilis

Toxic Shock Syndrome

Tuberculosis

Typhoid Fever

West Nile Virus

DEADLY DISEASES AND EPIDEMICS

MENINGITIS

Brian R. Shmaefsky

CONSULTING EDITOR
The Late I. **Edward Alcamo**
The Late Distinguished Teaching Professor of Microbiology,
SUNY Farmingdale

FOREWORD BY
David Heymann
World Health Organization

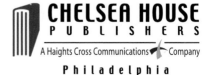

CHELSEA HOUSE
P U B L I S H E R S
A Haights Cross Communications Company

Philadelphia

Cover: Scanning electron micrograph of *Listeria monocytogenes*, one of the types of bacteria that cause meningitis.

Dedication
We dedicate the books in the DEADLY DISEASES AND EPIDEMICS series to Ed Alcamo, whose wit, charm, intelligence, and commitment to biology education were second to none.

CHELSEA HOUSE PUBLISHERS
VP, NEW PRODUCT DEVELOPMENT Sally Cheney
DIRECTOR OF PRODUCTION Kim Shinners
CREATIVE MANAGER Takeshi Takahashi
MANUFACTURING MANAGER Diann Grasse

Staff for Meningitis
EXECUTIVE EDITOR Tara Koellhoffer
ASSOCIATE EDITOR Beth Reger
PRODUCTION EDITOR Noelle Nardone
PHOTO EDITOR Sarah Bloom
SERIES DESIGNER Terry Mallon
COVER DESIGNER Keith Trego
LAYOUT 21st Century Publishing and Communications, Inc.

http://www.chelseahouse.com

First Printing

1 3 5 7 9 8 6 4 2

Library of Congress Cataloging-in-Publication Data

Shmaefsky, Brian.
    Meningitis/Brian R. Shmaefsky; foreword by David Heymann.
    p. cm.—(Deadly diseases and epidemics)
Includes bibliographical references and index.
    ISBN 0-7910-6701-7   0-7910-8344-6 (pbk.)
    1. Meningitis. I. Title. II. Series.
RC124.S54 2004
616.8'2—dc22

                                                        2004016201

All links and web addresses were checked and verified to be correct at the time of publication. Because of the dynamic nature of the web, some addresses and links may have changed since publication and may no longer be valid.

WITHDRAWN

Table of Contents

Foreword

In the 1960s, many of the infectious diseases that had terrorized generations were tamed. After a century of advances, the leading killers of Americans both young and old were being prevented with new vaccines or cured with new medicines. The risk of death from pneumonia, tuberculosis (TB), meningitis, influenza, whooping cough, and diphtheria declined dramatically. New vaccines lifted the fear that summer would bring polio, and a global campaign was on the verge of eradicating smallpox worldwide. New pesticides like DDT cleared mosquitoes from homes and fields, thus reducing the incidence of malaria, which was present in the southern United States and which remains a leading killer of children worldwide. New technologies produced safe drinking water and removed the risk of cholera and other water-borne diseases. Science seemed unstoppable. Disease seemed destined to all but disappear.

But the euphoria of the 1960s has evaporated.

The microbes fought back. Those causing diseases like TB and malaria evolved resistance to cheap and effective drugs. The mosquito developed the ability to defuse pesticides. New diseases emerged, including AIDS, Legionnaires, and Lyme disease. And diseases which had not been seen in decades re-emerged, as the hantavirus did in the Navajo Nation in 1993. Technology itself actually created new health risks. The global transportation network, for example, meant that diseases like West Nile virus could spread beyond isolated regions and quickly become global threats. Even modern public health protections sometimes failed, as they did in 1993 in Milwaukee, Wisconsin, resulting in 400,000 cases of the digestive system illness cryptosporidiosis. And, more recently, the threat from smallpox, a disease believed to be completely eradicated, has returned along with other potential bioterrorism weapons such as anthrax.

The lesson is that the fight against infectious diseases will never end.

In our constant struggle against disease, we as individuals have a weapon that does not require vaccines or drugs, and that is the warehouse of knowledge. We learn from the history of science that "modern" beliefs can be wrong. In this series of books, for example, you will learn that diseases like syphilis were once thought to be caused by eating potatoes. The invention of the microscope set science on the right path. There are more positive lessons from history. For example, smallpox was eliminated by vaccinating everyone who had come in contact with an infected person. This "ring" approach to smallpox control is still the preferred method for confronting an outbreak, should the disease be intentionally reintroduced.

At the same time, we are constantly adding new drugs, new vaccines, and new information to the warehouse. Recently, the entire human genome was decoded. So too was the genome of the parasite that causes malaria. Perhaps by looking at the microbe and the victim through the lens of genetics we will be able to discover new ways to fight malaria, which remains the leading killer of children in many countries.

Because of advances in our understanding of such diseases as AIDS, entire new classes of anti-retroviral drugs have been developed. But resistance to all these drugs has already been detected, so we know that AIDS drug development must continue.

Education, experimentation, and the discoveries that grow out of them are the best tools to protect health. Opening this book may put you on the path of discovery. I hope so, because new vaccines, new antibiotics, new technologies, and, most importantly, new scientists are needed now more than ever if we are to remain on the winning side of this struggle against microbes.

David Heymann
Executive Director
Communicable Diseases Section
World Health Organization
Geneva, Switzerland

Preface and Dedication

Diseases of the central nervous system can have unexpected effects on a person. Physicians have learned about the way the brain works by studying patients with central nervous system damage. The most common studies about brain function investigated the effects of strokes on behavior and movement. Stroke involves an interuption of blood flow to specific regions of the brain. Studies of stroke victims revealed that the ability to recognize an object is divided up among various regions of the brain. For example, the memory of seeing an apple is stored in a different part of brain from the memories of hearing the word *apple*, spelling the word *apple*, and tasting an *apple*. Strokes to a small region of the brain could cause a person to know the word apple and even be aware of the fruit's taste without being able to visualize an apple. Studies of people with the degenerative brain disorder Alzheimer's disease revealed that the condition causes people to lose specific memories while other memories remain intact. Investigating the effects of spinal cord injuries and infectious diseases such as encephalitis and meningitis has also contributed to our knowledge of brain function. Immune system chemicals that disrupt neuron communication cause the hallucinations—illusions of feeling, hearing, or seeing something that does not exist—that result from many types of meningitis. It is believed that too much or too little stimulation to nerves creates hallucinations. The aggressive and irritable behaviors attributed to rabies reflect cell damage by the viral attack. Disturbances in brain functions caused by chemical imbalances usually disappear after the disease is gone. However, brain damage due to dead or injured neurons and neuroglia is usually permanent. In some instances, other parts of the brain can take over for lost functions.

This book is dedicated to the memory of David Shmaefsky, also known as Daveed Schmayevski ben Samuél. In 1981, he lost a prolonged battle against nervous system damage precipitated by a stroke.

Brian R. Shmaefsky
Kingwood College

1

Panic–The Silent Epidemic

On January 24, 2001, the two top stories that appeared in the *East Montgomery County Observer* (a Texas newspaper) led with the headlines: "Thousands Get Vaccinated Against Meningitis" and "Outbreak Hits HISD." (HISD refers to Humble Independent School District in north suburban Houston.) The first headline described the fear unleashed upon a community by several critical cases and one fatality from the disease meningitis among school-age children in the region. The second headline reflected a misunderstanding of the epidemiological term *outbreak*. Both headlines heralded a concern that had long been ignored by public health agencies—the concern that children and young adults in schools, colleges, and the military are particularly susceptible to various forms of meningitis. Unfortunately, it took the death of a young person to bring public awareness to this problem.

Cases of meningitis started showing up across the 65-mile stretch of greater metropolitan Houston in January 2001, during the peak of cold and flu season. The *East Montgomery County Observer* and other newspapers serving nearby communities gave front-page coverage to each case of meningitis in the region. This publicity set in motion a flurry of activity to quell public fears. First came a mass vaccination campaign carried out by the Humble Independent School District. Several schools in the district set up free vaccination clinics for students. To handle the large numbers of students in the district, vaccinations were scheduled to be administered over a three-day period. Fearful parents who did not want to wait for their child's scheduled day overwhelmed local physicians' offices with requests for vaccinations. The supply of **vaccine** soon fell short, causing many panicked people to travel to other parts of Texas or to nearby states for vaccination.

Because of the activity in the Humble area, other local school districts felt compelled to set up their own vaccination programs. School boards were in a quandary, wondering whether it was necessary to provide vaccinations for their students. Some school officials worried that their students could develop a fatal case of meningitis if all or most of the students were not vaccinated. Others were concerned that many children could become ill from a vaccination that was really not needed. New Caney Independent School District, located a few miles north of Humble, voted to put a vaccination plan in place for its 10,000 students. The decision came about after adamant parents put pressure on the district that included protests and petitions to public health agencies. None of the schools or public health agencies in the area was prepared to deal with the apparent outbreak of meningitis. John Widmier, an assistant superintendent in the Humble Independent School District, summarized the situation in a *Humble Observer* newspaper article, stating, "We basically started with a blank slate"—meaning that the schools had no plan in place prior to the disease outbreak.

The lack of preparedness to deal with disease outbreaks abruptly appeared in the national news in the fall of 2001, when a suspicious occurrence of the rare disease **anthrax** infected 22 people and caused the death of 5. Anthrax is a disease caused by *Bacillus anthracis*, a bacterium that spreads easily from person to person and may cause severe internal bleeding. This outbreak appeared to be a bioterrorism attack in which anthrax-containing letters were mailed to influential media and government officials. The U.S. government learned quickly that few plans were in place to handle a bioterrorism attack that used deadly microorganisms such as anthrax.

As deadly as it can be, however, anthrax is easier to detect and to control than meningitis. First, anthrax produces a set of conditions that is likely to be associated with the particular organisms that cause the disease. In contrast, the conditions leading to meningitis vary greatly. Meningitis can start out as a mild condition that is difficult to detect or can begin as a severe disease that kills the afflicted person even before it is diagnosed. In addition, a person carrying the disease organism that causes anthrax will most likely get the disease and spread it to other people. This is not true for meningitis. The microorganisms that cause meningitis are present in most people and can spread without detection. To make the situation even more complicated, most people who carry the microorganisms that cause meningitis never come down with the disease. The microorganisms usually travel undetected from one person to another, making it very hard to predict where and when the disease will spread.

MENINGITIS: MANY DISEASES IN ONE

Meningitis is an **inflammation** of a **membrane,** called the **meninges,** that covers the brain and spinal cord. Damage to the meninges produces a variety of problems, ranging from a high fever with headaches to unconsciousness and death. Unfortunately for physicians, each case of meningitis is different. As we will see, various types of bacteria, viruses, fungi, and protozoa—many of which live normally in the body—are known to cause meningitis. This not only makes the disease challenging to diagnose, but also complicates the physician's ability to determine how it will affect the patient. The successful treatment of any disease depends on the physician's ability to determine how it will affect the patient. Without this information, it is difficult to know which medications are needed and what procedures should be done to counteract complications.

DOES THE MEDIA HELP OR HINDER?

Why does it appear that the news media overreact to many issues in our daily lives? Sometimes, it seems that much of the information in the news is blown out of proportion. This was the sentiment of many people who were reading about and listening to coverage of the meningitis scare in the Houston area in 2001. Public health officials had mixed feelings about the media exposure given to the meningitis crisis. The front-page coverage given to each case of meningitis packed medical centers and physicians' offices with panicked parents trying to get vaccinations for their children. Vaccine supplies quickly ran out. Many people who were not at risk for meningitis ended up getting vaccinated, while others who really needed the vaccine had trouble finding it.

There was, however, a positive side to the media coverage. It brought about an awareness of the dangers of bacterial meningitis. Many of the follow-up stories had educational aspects. Schools used the widespread publicity to start up meningitis prevention programs for students. The programs focused on the proper sanitation required for controlling meningitis and other contagious bacterial diseases. Nearby colleges also promoted meningitis awareness. Today's usual approach to news coverage is intended to goad the public to act on issues. The days of merely presenting information are gone. Those who report the news see public reaction to the media—for good or for bad—as a way to tell whether they are doing their job well.

Diseases that are difficult to predict and that appear without warning cause what scientists call silent outbreaks. The term **outbreak** refers to the rapid spread of a disease among many people living within a certain area. The newspapers in the Houston area called the cases of meningitis appearing in the nearby schools an outbreak because the disease showed up in 10 students within a week. Other cases started to emerge throughout Houston, making it look as though the disease were spreading through the whole region. Eventually, by a month after the first cases were detected, 40 cases of meningitis were confirmed across the metropolitan area. More startling to the public was that the disease seemed to pop up unexpectedly and randomly throughout distant regions of Houston. Nobody was able to predict where it would appear next. It seemed that the area was dealing with a silent outbreak.

To qualify as an outbreak, at least 10 people in a population of 100,000 must come down with the disease within a three-week period. Montgomery County had a population of 190,432 people at the time that the meningitis cases started appearing. Only 14 cases were confirmed within a three-week period. The 40 cases covering Montgomery County and Harris County cropped up in a population of almost 3.5 million people. That meant that the number of cases was well below the level that would be considered a true outbreak.

Even though the meningitis cases in the Houston metropolitan area did not qualify as an "official" outbreak, they nonetheless raised a number of legitimate concerns about controlling the spread of deadly diseases. First, how can a community prepare for a disease that emerges without warning? Second, how is it possible to predict the spread of a disease that has many causes? Third, how do physicians prepare to treat patients for a disease that is caused by organisms that live naturally in all humans? Fourth, how should private citizens and public agencies be alerted about a disease that has a wide variety of characteristics? Fifth, how does the medical community care for a large population of people in a situation where a disease—like meningitis— requires a variety of treatments? The 2001 meningitis scare made scientists think seriously about how best to answer all these questions.

2

Meningitis–Attack on the Nervous System

Veni, vidi, vici (I came, I saw, I conquered).
—Julius Caesar, Roman ruler, 100–44 B.C.

Julius Caesar's statement describing the swift success of his Roman army in a battle in Anatolia in 47 B.C. could just as effectively be used to describe the **microorganisms** that invade the nervous system. Various types of bacteria, viruses, fungi, and protozoa are capable of causing some degree of nervous system damage (which may or may not be permanent). Although the nervous system is one of the toughest body components for microorganisms to invade, some microorganisms can indeed conquer it, leading—as we will learn later—to diseases called meningitis, **encephalitis**, and **meningoencephalitis.**

The body is normally home to many types of microorganisms that live on the skin and the inner mucous membrane surfaces of the digestive system, reproductive tract, respiratory system, and urinary tract. Note that the microorganisms are generally on the body surfaces and not actually inside of the body. These organisms usually cause little or no harm to people. In fact, many of the bacteria and fungi on the skin and in the mucous membranes prevent **pathogens**, organisms that cause disease, from gaining ground in the body. Other bacteria and fungi in the digestive system help break down food and provide nutrients that are not normally available through the diet. Unlike the rest of the body, however, the nervous system is not home to any microorganisms.

If microorganisms do gain access to the nervous system, the result is damage to the nerve cells.

Infectious diseases of the nervous system (Figure 2.1) are very rare. But when these diseases do occur, they usually cause great harm that can lead to permanent impairment or death. However, in order to cause harm to the nervous system, microorganisms must first pass through the body's defenses and find their way to the nervous system, which is buried deep in the body tissues. The degree of damage caused by microorganisms depends on which portion of the nervous system is under attack. For example, injury to the brain has a greater impact on a person than damage to a nerve that just controls a finger.

CELLS OF THE NERVOUS SYSTEM

A view through a microscope reveals that the nervous system is made up of two types of cells: neurons and neuroglial cells. **Neurons** (Figure 2.2) are the cells that send information from one part of the body to another. Heat, sight, smell, and touch are some examples of the types of communication passed along by neurons. Neurons produce chemicals called **neurotransmitters** to send information from one neuron to another. Neurons also use neurotransmitters to control body organs. For example, neurons use these chemical messengers to control how muscles flex and how the digestive system breaks down food.

Neurotransmitters send information to neurons by turning on an electric charge in a nerve impulse. The **nerve impulse** helps neurons pass along the information to other neurons or body cells. Neurons must be free of disease in order to respond to neurotransmitters and pass along the information using the nerve impulse. Neurons located in organs called **sensory structures** produce nerve impulses after they receive information from the environment. Instead of responding to internal neurotransmitters, they react to chemicals, light, and pressure. Chemicals that come in contact with the sensory structures of the tongue produce taste. Light

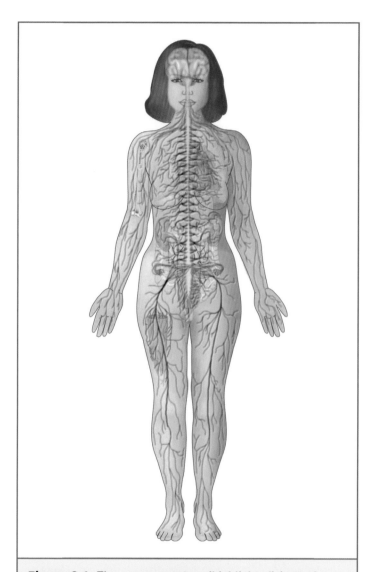

Figure 2.1 The nervous system (highlighted) is rarely infected by viruses or bacteria, but when it is, the results can be deadly. Luckily, the central nervous system in particular is well protected from infection by a covering called the meninges and special blood vessels called the blood-brain barrier. Infections of any part of the nervous system can lead to a loss of important bodily functions.

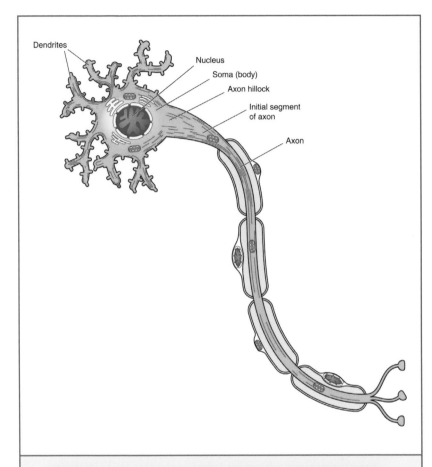

Dendrites

Nucleus

Soma (body)

Axon hillock

Initial segment
of axon

Axon

Figure 2.2 A neuron, illustrated here, is a nerve cell that sends
information from one part of the body to another. Neurons receive
messages through branch-like dendrites, and transmit those signals to
other cells through the axon (the long "tail" coming off the neuron's
cell body). The signals are then passed to another neuron by special
chemicals called neurotransmitters.

that enters the sensory structures of the eye produces sight.
Pressure to the sensory structures of the skin allows the
feeling of touch. Again, it is important to remember that only
healthy sensory structures are able to send information from
the environment to neurons.

Neuroglial cells are the other type of cell making up the nervous system. They protect neurons and help them function. There is a different type of neuroglial cell for each function. The most common type of neuroglial cell is called a **Schwann cell**. These cells wrap around neurons, helping the neuron produce faster impulses. Without Schwann cells, the nervous system would react very slowly, if at all. Aside from helping with impulses, scientists have discovered that Schwann cells also help damaged neurons heal. Other types of neuroglial cells protect neurons from disease and poisons. Neurons would quickly die without the assistance of these cells.

ANATOMY OF THE NERVOUS SYSTEM

Neurons and neuroglial cells work together to create the nervous system. Neurons are bundled together into large structures called nerves. **Nerves** carry large amounts of information for the nervous system. In almost all animals, the nervous system consists of two parts: the **peripheral nervous system** and the **central nervous system** (Figure 2.3). The peripheral system is made up of nerves that run throughout the body. These peripheral nerves can be found underneath the skin, in each body organ, and around all the muscles. They carry out two functions: to pass information from the body to the brain, and to bring information from the brain to the rest of the body.

Sensory nerves in the peripheral nervous system carry information from the body to the brain. These nerves receive messages from skin, muscles, and organs through special nerve cells called **sensory receptors**. The sensory receptors detect information such as balance, hearing, sight, smell, and touch. Without receptors, the body would not know what is going on in the outside environment. Diseases of the sensory receptors or nerves prevent certain kinds of information from going to the brain. Certain bacterial diseases of skin, such as leprosy, cause a loss of pain, temperature detection, and touch in the skin. People with leprosy are very likely to damage their

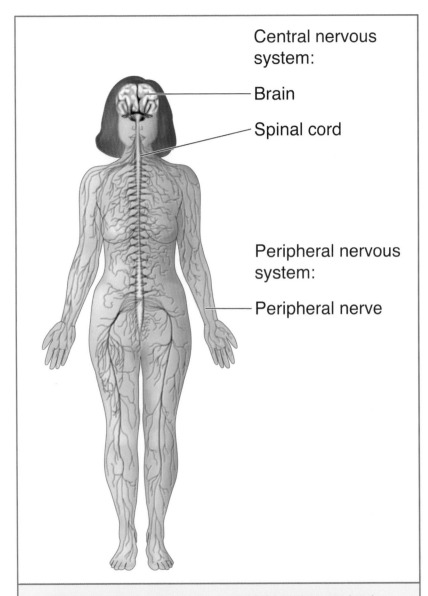

Central nervous system:

Brain

Spinal cord

Peripheral nervous system:

Peripheral nerve

Figure 2.3 The nervous system is divided into the central and peripheral nervous systems. The peripheral nervous system is composed of nerves that run to all areas of the body. The central nervous system is made up of the brain and spinal cord, and controls all of the other nerves in the body.

hands and even accidentally cut off a finger without realizing they have harmed themselves.

Motor nerves in the peripheral nervous system carry information from the brain to the body. Scientists came up with the name "motor" because the first motor nerves studied were those that help with muscle movement, or what scientists call **motor function**. It was later discovered that motor nerves have other purposes in addition to making muscles move. They also send messages from the brain and the spinal cord to body organs. For example, motor nerves help the process of digestion by stimulating cells in the stomach to break down food chemically. Motor nerve damage can leave a person unable to move a body part or incapable of controlling an organ. Automobile accidents and falls are common causes of motor nerve injury. However, several types of bacteria and viruses can also permanently destroy motor nerves. A viral disease called polio spread throughout America and Europe in the early 20th century. It left many people unable to move their limbs or even their entire bodies. This condition, known as **paralysis**, even made it impossible for some victims of polio to breathe because the nerves going to muscles in the chest were not able to function unaided.

Motor and sensory nerves serve one of two divisions of the peripheral nervous system: the **somatic nervous system** and the **autonomic nervous system**. The somatic nervous system is often considered voluntary, because it is, for the most part, subject to conscious control by the brain. Somatic nerves go to the skin and muscles, allowing the body to sense and respond to pain, temperature, and touch. Being poked by a sharp object stimulates the somatic nervous system. Both the pain and the rapid body movement that results as a response to being poked are due to the actions of sensory and motor nerves in the somatic nervous system.

The autonomic nervous system is considered involuntary, because it has automatic control over many body organs.

Balance, heart rate, respiration, digestion, hearing, and vision are all under automatic control. Two different types of nerve tracts make up the autonomic nervous system: the parasympathetic nervous system and the sympathetic nervous system. The **parasympathetic nervous system** puts the body at rest and helps with the digestion of food. Neurotransmitters from parasympathetic nerves slow down the heart and lungs, and decrease blood flow to the muscles. At the same time, they increase blood flow to the digestive organs and stimulate digestive tract secretions.

The effect of the **sympathetic nervous system** on the body is opposite to that of the parasympathetic. For example, the sympathetic nervous system prepares the body for action by directing blood flow to the muscles, giving them the nutrients and oxygen they need to perform activities such as running or hard physical labor. Sympathetic nerves speed up the heart and lungs, helping the body keep up with increased activity, and stimulate the sweat glands that help cool the body. Diseases of the autonomic nervous system are usually very serious, if not deadly. They generally affect many body functions, leaving the body unable to adapt to changes in its internal environment.

THE CENTRAL NERVOUS SYSTEM

The peripheral nervous system can carry out some tasks on its own. However, most of its commands come from the central nervous system. The central nervous system is composed of the brain and spinal cord (refer again to Figure 2.3 on page 21).

The **brain**, a complicated collection of neurons and neuroglial cells, controls almost all of the nervous system. It is the biggest and most sophisticated part of the central nervous system. The brain is divided into a large section called the cerebrum and a small section behind the cerebrum called the cerebellum. The **cerebrum** coordinates most of the nervous system's functions. It is composed of sections called lobes.

Each lobe carries out a different brain function. For example, the temporal lobe, located just behind the ears, assists in hearing and speech. The capacity to concentrate on thoughts and the ability to coordinate movements such as writing and walking are controlled by the frontal lobe, located at the front of the cerebrum. Hidden behind the cerebrum is the **cerebellum**, which coordinates complex body movements, such as balance. Destruction of either the neurons or neuroglial cells of the brain cause a loss of the particular functions associated with the specific region damaged.

The **brain stem** is an area of the brain connecting the cerebrum and cerebellum to the spinal cord. It is composed of various regions that interpret and organize information coming from the peripheral nervous system. In addition, the brain stem controls many automatic functions of the central nervous system. Breathing rate, heart rate, hunger, sleep, and thirst are all regulated by the brain stem. The brain stem also works with the cerebellum to handle complicated body movements. The activities of walking up a staircase while simultaneously carrying a handful of books and talking to friends are synchronized by the brain stem working together with the cerebrum and cerebellum. Many types of diseases can cause damage to the brain stem. Injury to the brain stem is similar to damage to the brain. The specific effect on the body depends on where precisely the damage occurred.

Underneath the brain stem lies the **spinal cord**, a long bundle of nerves that runs down the length of the body. Its main job is to carry information between the brain stem and the peripheral nervous system. The spinal cord connects to the peripheral nervous system with 31 pairs of spinal nerves. Each spinal nerve communicates with a specific part of the body. Spinal nerves coming from the neck transfer information to the lower head, neck, and shoulders. **Reflexes**, automatic responses to something that stimulates the body, are controlled by the spinal cord. Physicians use reflexes to diagnose damage

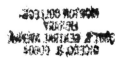

to the spinal cord. For example, a sharp tap to the knee causes a knee jerk reflex. If a person is unable to produce this reflex, it may mean there is damage to spinal nerves of the lower back.

Covering the central nervous system are three layers of tissue that are collectively called the meninges (Figure 2.4). Above that, the skull and vertebral column form a bone covering that protects the meninges and underlying nervous system from injury. Each of the three layers of the meninges has a particular function in protecting the brain and spinal cord. The outermost layer, the **dura mater**, is a thick covering that contains blood vessels, a layer of fat, and nerves. The dura mater cushions the central nervous system, keeping it from knocking into the skull and vertebral column. It is also a barrier that prevents infectious microorganisms from invading the underlying neurons and neuroglial cells.

Below the dura mater is a layer of meninges called the **arachnoid mater**. This layer gets its name from the scientific term for spiders (*arachnid*), because, under a microscope, it looks like a spiderweb. The delicate arachnoid layer forms a subarachnoid space that contains the **cerebrospinal fluid**, a protective secretion that cushions the central nervous system. Cerebral spinal fluid flows from the arachnoid layer to cavities and canals in the brain stem and spinal cord.

The innermost layer of the meninges is a very thin membrane called the **pia mater**. Like the dura mater, it contains blood vessels and nerves. Its function is to nourish the neurons and neuroglial cells of the central nervous system. The pia mater also protects the central nervous system from many toxic chemicals and microorganisms that enter the blood.

Damage to the meninges causes a type of inflammation called meningitis. Falls or impact injuries that bruise the meninges are one cause of meningitis. It is not unusual to find this type of meningitis associated with automobile accidents and war wounds. This type of meningitis can heal quickly and seldom causes long-term damage to the central nervous system.

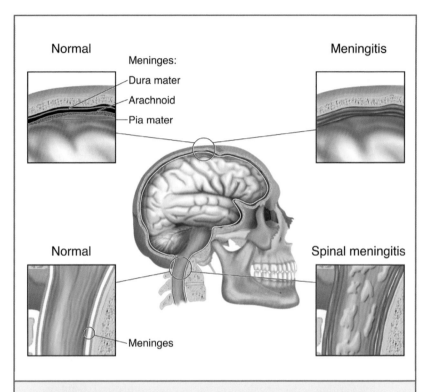

Figure 2.4 The central nervous system (spinal cord and brain) is covered by layers of tissue called meninges. There are three layers of meninges—the dura mater, the pia mater, and the arachnoid, which contain cerebrospinal fluid to cushion the other structures. Meningitis occurs when bacteria, viruses, or other foreign organisms invade and infect the cerebrospinal fluid, causing the meninges to swell and become inflamed.

Brain and spinal cord cancers can also lead to meningitis. These are difficult to treat and are very destructive to the central nervous system. Attacks on the nervous system from bacteria and viruses, discussed in the following chapters, can also cause meningitis. In many instances, this type of meningitis can cause permanent central nervous system damage or death. Unfortunately, the body has few ways to defend the meninges against infectious disease once microorganisms have made their way into the central nervous system. The meninges rely on body defenses in the mucous membranes, skin, and blood for protection against invasion by microorganisms.

THE BLOOD-BRAIN BARRIER

Most animals have a simple central nervous system made up of neuron groupings called ganglia. Ganglia work together to carry out simple tasks that help the organism survive. Insects and worms rely on this type of nervous system. Larger animals, such as fish and frogs, have neuroglial cells to better organize and speed up the actions of the central nervous system. They have also developed the membranes known as meninges to protect the central nervous system. Mammals added another layer of complexity to the central nervous system. They have what scientists call the **blood-brain barrier**. The blood-brain barrier is not a single identifiable structure. It is a combination of blood vessels and neuroglial cells that protect the brain from damage caused by chemicals or microbes. Thin blood vessels called capillaries form tightly sealed tubes that let only nutrients and wastes flow between the blood and the brain. Neuroglial cells called astrocytes take away any toxins that may injure the brain.

Many medical students perform a simple experiment that shows the value of the blood-brain barrier. They inject a live rat with a blue dye that stains cells. After circulating throughout the body, the dye stains all the cells of the rat except those in the central nervous system. This is because the blood-brain barrier blocks the dye from going to the brain. This experiment also illustrates an important feature of the blood-brain barrier. While protecting the brain from undesirable elements, it also blocks antibiotics and other medications from getting to the central nervous system. To counter this problem when they need to treat a brain infection, physicians must inject the medications directly into the cerebrospinal fluid.

THE IMMUNE SYSTEM FIGHTS BACK

The various types of infectious meningitis belong to a group of diseases called septic diseases, or septicemias. **Septicemia** refers to the presence of microorganisms in the bloodstream. The bacteria, fungi, protista, and viruses that cause meningitis must pass into the bloodstream to attach the meninges. Normally, the blood is free of microorganisms—including bacteria, fungi, and protozoa—that can only be seen with a microscope. However, microorganisms sometimes make their way into the bloodstream. When they do this, they always cause disease. The illness associated with septicemia is caused by two conditions: bacterial secretions and an over-response of the immune system to the microbial invasion. **Secretions** are substances that flow out of cells or microorganisms. Secretions produced by the cells of the body's immune system can cause fever, rashes, and fatigue. Similarly, secretions made by the microorganisms themselves produce a variety of disease signs and symptoms. Physicians define a **sign** as a condition that can be measured or seen by the doctor. Redness, sores, and swelling are examples of disease signs. The term **symptom** refers to a subjective condition felt by the patient. Dizziness, headache, nausea, and pain are examples of disease symptoms. The microorganisms that cause meningitis can produce some or all of these conditions in people.

The body's **immune system** (Figure 2.5), the complex system of body organs and cells that help recognize and fight off disease, has two ways to prevent the spread of microorganisms throughout the blood. Its first strategy is to stop microorganisms from entering the body in the first place. The second method attempts to kill and remove any microorganisms that do manage to enter. The form of immunity called nonspecific immunity can be divided into three components: physical barriers, chemical deterrents, and cellular attack. Chemical deterrents and physical barriers form the first line of defense, using the skin and body linings to act as walls that prevent microorganisms from invading.

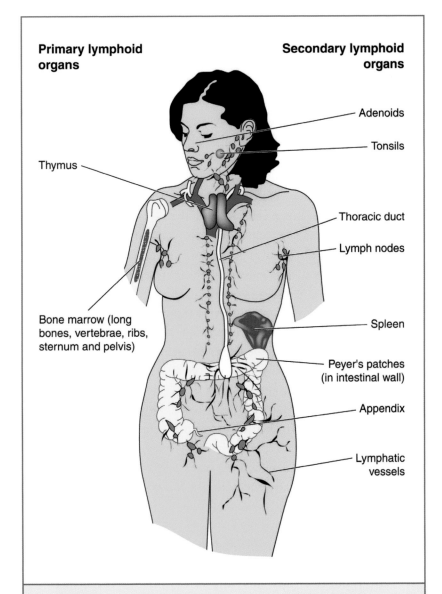

Primary lymphoid organs

Secondary lymphoid organs

Adenoids

Tonsils

Thymus

Thoracic duct

Lymph nodes

Bone marrow (long bones, vertebrae, ribs, sternum and pelvis)

Spleen

Peyer's patches (in intestinal wall)

Appendix

Lymphatic vessels

Figure 2.5 The immune system protects the body from injury and disease, and fights foreign organisms that breach its outer defenses. The parts of the immune system are sometimes referred to as lymphoid organs. The various components of the immune system are illustrated here.

Skin and **mucous membranes**, the moist mucus-covered tissue that lines the digestive, respiratory, reproductive, and urinary systems, compose the body's physical barriers. They work to prevent invasion by microorganisms. Mucous membranes and skin form a continuous sheet of cells that surround the body and line its organs. This lining blocks invasion of the blood and internal organs, and stops most of the microorganisms that cause meningitis. Unfortunately, some of the microorganisms that cause meningitis can get past this barrier. They produce secretions that break down the tight connections between cells, making the barrier useless until it heals or defends itself in other ways. Some of the organisms that cause meningitis can get past this barrier when they are injected into the body by animal bites.

Mucus—a thick, sticky fluid produced by the mucous membranes—also physically removes microorganisms. The sticky mucus secreted by the respiratory system continuously moves upward from the lungs to the throat. This keeps microorganisms from entering the body through the delicate membranes of the lungs. Mucus is also present in the digestive system, reproductive tract, and urinary tract. It prevents microorganisms from sticking to the body cells and helps flush them out of the body. Almost all microorganisms cling to mucus, making it a good mechanism for clearing the body of organisms that cause meningitis. Unfortunately, this barrier does not prevent the invasion of microorganisms introduced into the body by animal bites.

Oily skin secretions, sweat, tears, urine, and digestive enzymes are the body's chemical deterrents. Microorganisms have a difficult time surviving in the oily secretions and sweat produced by the skin. Oils produced by **sebaceous glands** prevent microorganisms from sticking to the skin, making them easier to wash away. Sweat contains acids and salts that inhibit the growth of bacteria and fungi on the skin. Enzymes in the sweat degrade many viruses that make contact with skin. This then keeps down the population of microorganisms that live on the skin. Too large a population of microorganisms on the skin increases the chance that they could accidentally enter the body through wounds. Tears and urine reduce the growth of microorganisms by flushing them from the body. Tears remove microorganisms from the eyes, while urine flushes out the urinary tract, and also contains enzymes that stop the growth of microorganisms. Digestive enzymes in the stomach and intestines are able to destroy many microorganisms that can invade the body through the digestive system.

Chemical barriers traveling in the blood attempt to break apart, poison, or starve microorganisms that do make their way into the body. There are at least a dozen proteins in the blood that help remove microorganisms from the body. They also produce the fever, inflammation, and other signs associated with septic diseases such as meningitis. A large group of proteins making up the complement system attach to micro-organisms, ultimately killing them or helping blood cells to remove them. Chemicals called **interferons** mostly target viruses. Interferons keep viruses from infecting body cells and help get rid of cells that are being attacked by viruses. Chemical secretions called **necrotic factors** discourage large microorganisms such as fungi, protozoa, and worms. Necrotic factors break down microorganisms by poking holes in their cells.

A group of cells roaming the body and floating in the blood make up the second line of defense of nonspecific immunity. These cells are stimulated by many of the secre-tions produced for the chemical defense. Large cells called **macrophages** travel around the body destroying microorgan-isms. They are found on body linings, throughout various tissues, and in the blood. Macrophages in the body linings prevent microorganisms from entering the body. Those found in the tissues and blood attack microorganisms that manage to pass into the body. Macrophages are very effective at removing the bacteria and fungi that cause meningitis. Other cells called **lymphocytes** make up an early warning system that tells the body about an invasion by microbes (microorganisms). Lymphocyte secretions usually stimulate other immune system cells. Some of these secretions help other cells fend off viruses. Cells called **eosinophils** and **neutrophils** also assist with the early warning system by signaling other cells about invading microorganisms. In addition, they produce secretions that mount a chemical defense. The fever associated with meningitis is due to cellular secretions called cytokines. **Fever** is not a negative consequence of the disease, but rather a method of killing septic microorganisms. The elevated body temperature produced during fever inhibits the metabolism of microorganisms, causing them to die off more readily.

Specific immunity is another immune system strategy for killing microorganisms that enter the body. It carries out this task by mounting a specific attack that targets only the microorganism that causes the disease. Specific immunity reduces an ongoing invasion and supplies the body with a way to act more quickly in the event of subsequent attacks by the same invader. Unlike nonspecific immunity, specific immunity improves with exposure to the disease and makes sure that future attacks are quickly resisted. Specific immunity begins when a microorganism enters the body after getting past the nonspecific defenses. A macrophage finds and engulfs the microorganism. Digested components of the microorganism called **antigens** are then placed on the surface of the macrophage. This macrophage then travels to cells called lymphocytes, which are found in lymphatic tissue. A lymphocyte called a **T helper cell** then attaches to the antigen on the macrophage, which alerts the immune system that a particular microorganism is in the body. Next, the T helper cell binds to another lymphocyte, called a **B cell**. B cells secrete proteins called **antibodies** that stick to the surface of the microorganism. Antibodies let the body know an **infection** is taking place. This begins a series of events in which the immune system attempts to rapidly destroy and remove that particular microorganism. The B cells continue to circulate around the body for several years, carrying a "memory" of a particular disease.

Specific immunity is the best defense against the meningitis microorganisms that enter the body through animal bites. However, specific immunity loses its effectiveness if the microorganisms make their way to the nervous system, the network that receives information from the environment and sends information throughout the body. Unfortunately, the nervous system has little protection from the immune system. Once in the nervous system, microorganisms can cause harm with little impunity. This is why meningitis outbreaks are such a worry to physicians and public health officials. They know that the disease can do a great deal of damage to the nervous system before it is successfully treated. The fact that meningitis can hide from the immune system once it is in the nervous system also makes some treatments ineffective. Thus, meningitis must be caught early if doctors hope to deal with it effectively. Preventing the spread of meningitis is probably the best plan for combating this potentially fatal disease. However, this is not easy to do, because the disease travels silently through the human population.

3

Bacterial Meningitis

If thine enemy hunger, feed him; if he thirst, give him drink.
—Romans 12:20

It is almost as if the central nervous system follows the biblical advice of Romans 12:20 when it is under attack by bacteria. Invading bacteria gain nourishment from the central nervous system tissues as if the body had been instructed to care for them. In actuality, the body is not intentionally helping the bacteria. Rather, the central nervous system is not fully equipped to fight infection, which makes it unable to hinder bacterial activity. In addition, the way bacteria feed makes the central nervous system vulnerable to an unrelenting assault. Bacterial meningitis is deadlier than many other forms of meningitis and septic diseases. This is not just because bacteria cause severe damage to the central nervous system; much of the disease's destructiveness is due to the unrestrained growth of the bacteria themselves as they feed on the central nervous system.

Bacteria are a diverse group of primitive microscopic organisms. Their body is composed of only a single cell usually surrounded by a rigid covering called a cell wall (Figure 3.1). Most bacteria reproduce very rapidly, as long as they have plenty of food. Bacteria are referred to as **saprotrophs,** which means that they feed on decaying material. To do this, bacteria secrete digestive **enzymes,** proteins that carry out chemical reactions. The chemical reactions of digestion break food down into simple chemicals that the bacterial cells can use as nutrients.

It is these bacterial secretions that make meningitis a serious condition, damaging the delicate meninges that cover and protect the central

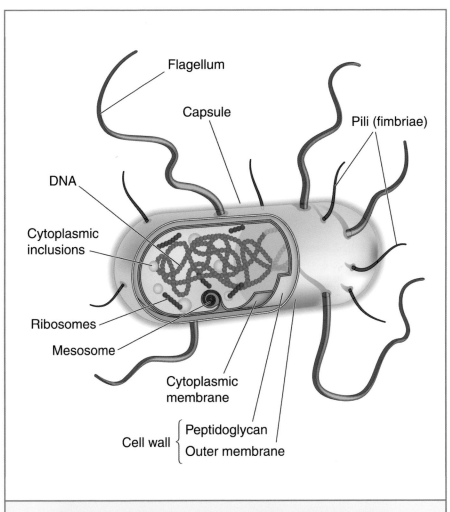

Figure 3.1 In general, bacteria are simple, prokaryotic cells. Most bacteria feed by breaking down dead animals and plants. However, some bacteria have the ability to dine on living organisms, causing illness and sometimes killing the organism.

nervous system. These secretions permit bacteria to kill the organism's living cells, which, in turn, become food for the bacteria. They also protect the bacteria from being removed by the body of the organism that has been invaded.

A bacterial attack of the body turns on a series of immune responses that harm both the body and the bacteria. This contributes (even if unwittingly) to the severity of the disease. All septic diseases pose this problem for physicians. Treatment has to take into account the damaging effects of both the bacteria and the body's immune system. Each requires a different strategy for reducing the destruction of bodily tissues. When the immune system itself causes damage to the body, this is referred to as **autoimmune disease**. Bacteria are noted for eliciting a strong autoimmune response in people. During bacterial meningitis, the meninges become inflamed partly as a result of immune system cell secretions. Early in meningitis, cells called lymphocytes stimulate the action of eosinophils and neutrophils. They secrete chemicals called cytokines that promote fever and blood flow. The increased blood flow causes swelling and reddening of the affected body part. Though the fever usually causes no damage, the swelling can put excessive pressure on the meninges, damaging the delicate membranes of the meninges and the underlying neurons and neuroglial cells.

Another source of damage during meningitis results from the activity of the B cells. B cells produce protein secretions called antibodies that bind to particular proteins on disease-causing organisms like bacteria. Unfortunately, the antibodies will sometimes bind to the surfaces of the meninges as well as to bacteria. Antibodies start a deadly response once they bind to proteins on the surfaces of cells. They stimulate a group of cells called cytotoxic (or killer) T cells. These cells produce necrotic factors that damage any nearby cells. Too much cytotoxic T cell activity will destroy body cells. Bacterial meningitis provokes a large cytotoxic T cell response, permitting the secretion of large amounts of necrotic factor that enters the cerebrospinal fluid and blood. Central nervous system damage occurs rapidly wherever necrotic factor is present. Unfortunately, the neurons and neuroglial cells have little protection against the body's production of necrotic factor.

Advanced bacterial meningitis is indicated by the presence of white blood cells in the cerebrospinal fluid. Normally, there are no blood cells of any type in the fluids of the central nervous system. Their presence always indicates damage or disease. Inflammation due to meningitis encourages certain white blood cells to enter the cerebrospinal fluid. One would think that their presence would help fight off disease, since that is what they do elsewhere in the body. However, the opposite is actually true. Their secretions do additional damage by killing body cells and leaving behind the decaying cells of bacteria. Dead cells cannot be replaced, and damaged neurons and neuroglial cells heal very slowly, if at all. As a result, the central nervous system can suffer permanent loss of a particular function.

BACTERIA THAT CAUSE MENINGITIS

Any bacterium that causes septic disease can produce meningitis. These bacteria attack other body organs as well as the central nervous system. The presence of bacteria in these organs means that they can make their way to the meninges. However, not all of them produce severe damage. The degree of damage depends on the types of secretions produced by the bacteria. Most of these bacteria live in the bodies of healthy people and never cause disease. Usually, the body's immune defenses keep the bacteria under control, preventing invasion and disease. However, other diseases, injury, or stress can weaken the immune system barriers. This leaves open an opportunity for the bacteria to invade the body and make their way into the bloodstream. Once in the bloodstream, the bacteria spread throughout the body and gain access to any organ, including the meninges. They can enter the meninges by traveling through the small blood vessels in the arachnoid mater and pia mater.

Three types of bacteria usually cause most cases of bacterial meningitis. They are *Haemophilus influenzae, Neisseria meningitidis,* and *Streptococcus pneumoniae.* All three types of bacteria are normal residents of the human respiratory system's mucous membranes. The bacteria are most commonly found in the nose, but they can make their way to the ears, eyes, and throat without causing disease. Their presence in other parts of the body, however, produces disease. All three of these bacteria more commonly cause diseases other than meningitis. In addition, they are all related to other bacteria that produce severe septic diseases.

Haemophilus influenzae

Microbiologists categorize *Haemophilus influenzae* as a gram-negative bacterium. Figure 3.2 shows a photograph of *H. influenzae* taken through a microscope. The gram-negative designation refers to a staining technique used to identify bacteria. Gram-negative bacteria appear purplish pink under a microscope. Knowing a bacterium's **Gram stain** designation is important for understanding how the bacterium causes disease. Gram-negative bacteria cause disease by secreting enzymes that digest the cells of the organism being invaded. Another important characteristic of gram-negative bacteria is their ability to release a group of very strong poisons called **endotoxins** when the cells are actively reproducing or upon cell death. Endotoxins cause extensive cell damage and stimulate autoimmune attack.

Haemophilus influenzae gets its name because microbiologists growing the bacterium in culture noted that it thrives on blood. The term *haemo* means "blood" and *philus* means "to love." Many parents are familiar with the childhood ear and eye infections caused by *H. influenzae.* **Conjunctivitis** (also called **pinkeye**) is one of the most common diseases the bacterium causes. However, the organism is also known to bring on respiratory infections resembling the

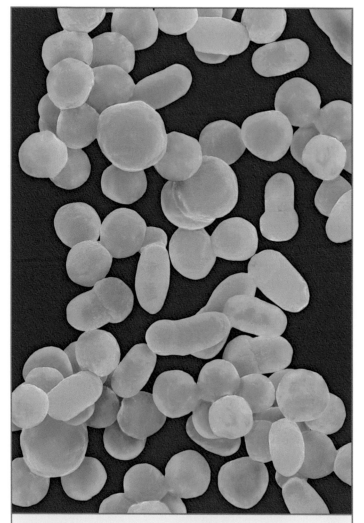

Figure 3.2 *Haemophilus influenzae*, shown here in purple among red blood cells, is a gram-negative bacterium that can cause meningitis, most commonly in young children.

flu; hence, the second part of the organism's name. Surprisingly, *H. influenzae* is normally found in the mucous membranes of most people. It is easily transferred from one person to another by coughing, sneezing, and touching. Children who do not wash their hands after touching their mouths or nose can pass along *H. influenzae* to their family members, friends, and classmates. Luckily, in most people, the bacterium causes no harm.

Meningitis due to *H. influenzae* is most common in children under 5 years of age. It was a major cause of meningitis in American children until vaccinations became common; it is now only prevalent in regions of world that do not vaccinate infants. Physicians discovered that a particular type of *H. influenzae* called Hib causes meningitis. **Hib** stands for *H. influenzae* type b. The "b" refers to a sugar-like chemical called a polysaccharide found on the surface of the bacterium. *H. influenzae* differs from many other bacteria because a protective layer called a capsule covers the bacteria's surface. The capsule prevents *H. influenzae* from drying out and allows it to stick to the surfaces of cells. Illnesses from *H. influenzae* begin when the organism starts to grow in large numbers and spreads outside the mucous membranes of the throat and nose. Large numbers of *H. influenzae* in the lower regions of the respiratory tract cause mucous membrane inflammation. Sometimes the bacteria are able to enter the bloodstream through irritated areas of the inflamed mucous membrane. Once in the bloodstream, *H. influenzae* can gain access to the meninges and cerebrospinal fluid.

Neisseria meningitidis

The name *Neisseria meningitidis* tells us that this bacterium is most noted for causing meningitis. It is not known to cause other diseases. *N. meningitidis* organisms live in the mucous membranes of many animals and are very common in the upper parts of the human respiratory system. Like *Haemophilus influenzae*, *Neisseria meningitidis* is a gram-negative bacterium, meaning that it, too, produces potent endotoxins. It differs from *Haemophilus influenzae* in that its cells are shaped like spheres (Figure 3.3). Spherical-shaped bacterial cells are called **cocci**. Thus, meningitis caused by *N. meningitidis* is called

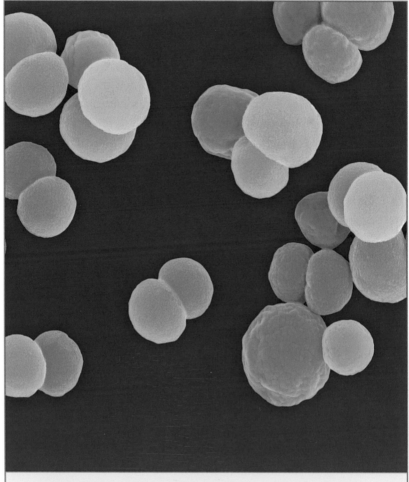

Figure 3.3 *Neisseria meningitidis* can cause meningitis. These bacteria cause a type of disease known as meningococcal meningitis, which is most common in infants. This photomicrograph was taken with a scanning electron microscope, magnified 3,750 times.

meningococcal meningitis. The bacteria require oxygen, so they prefer to live on body surfaces or areas in the body that are rich in oxygen. They can survive in blood and cerebrospinal fluid, however, because of the high amounts of oxygen carried in these fluids.

Meningococcal meningitis usually appears in children younger than one year old. However, it will occasionally show up in older children and adults. Because the bacterium lives in mucus, it is easily spread by coughing, sneezing, and touching. The bacterium very likely dies quickly when the mucus in which it resides dries. This means that it is not easily passed between people through hand contact or contact with surfaces such as tables, towels, and utensils. There are 12 different types of *N. meningitidis*, but only 5 strains can cause a fatal disease: types A, B, C, Y, and W135. These different strains make it difficult to create a meningitis vaccine. Vaccines usually work against only one particular strain of a disease.

Streptococcus pneumoniae

Approximately 60% of the pneumonia cases found in adults is due to *Streptococcus pneumoniae*. **Pneumonia** is a respiratory system infection that causes fluid buildup and inflammation in the lungs. What does this organism have to do with meningitis? The same bacterium can become septic and produce a disease called pneumococcal meningitis. *Streptococcus* is a large group of bacteria commonly found living on the skin and mucous membranes of many animals. Most types of *Streptococcus* actually are helpful in warding off **pathogenic** bacteria. However, some types cause disease if they grow too abundant or find their way past the body's barriers into the blood and internal organs. *Streptococcus pneumoniae* are very likely to cause disease because of their ability to invade the body. Some types of *S. pneumoniae* are more dangerous than others because of certain types of toxic secretions unique to certain groups of the bacteria. For example, some *Streptococcus* bacteria produce toxins called streptolysins while others do not. Streptolysins are proteins that cause red blood cells to break down. This produces a more serious condition because the red blood cells are needed to carry oxygen throughout the body.

Streptococcus that do not produce streptolysins cannot destroy red blood cells.

The name *Streptococcus* means "twisted chain." This term beautifully describes the microscopic view of this group of bacteria (Figure 3.4). The spherical cells of *Streptococcus* grow in long, twining chains. *Streptococcus* is a gram-positive bacterium, meaning that it causes illness by secreting a variety of exotoxins. **Exotoxins** are secretions released from the cell wall of bacteria that cause disease in the **host organism**. **Pyrogens** are a group of exotoxins that produce the intense fever characteristic of pneumococcal meningitis. Other exotoxins, including the pyrogens, produce a rash on the mucous membranes and skin (Figure 3.5). Exotoxins that produce a rash are called erythrogenic toxins. *Erythrogen* means "to turn red." Other *S. pneumoniae* secretions include a variety of enzymes that destroy host cells and tissues. **Hemolysins** are enzymes that destroy red blood cells, which provide an ample supply of the iron and protein needed for rapid *S. pneumoniae* growth. An enzyme called hyaluronidase helps *S. pneumoniae* digest its way through the body, permitting it to invade the blood and meninges readily. Deoxyribonuclease is secreted to assist with the digestion of **deoxyribonucleic acid** (**DNA**) from dying cells. Streptokinase is an enzyme unique to *S. pneumoniae* bacteria. It plays a special role in breaking down blood clots. This combats the body's ability to barricade the bacteria for destruction by white blood cells.

ORIGINS OF BACTERIAL MENINGITIS

Cattle farmers are all too familiar with bacteria that cause ear infections, pinkeye, and pneumonia in their livestock. Some of the same bacteria that produce these diseases in cattle— including *Haemophilus, Neisseria* and *Streptococcus*—cause similar diseases in humans. Scientists believe that wild animals suffered from diseases caused by these bacteria long before

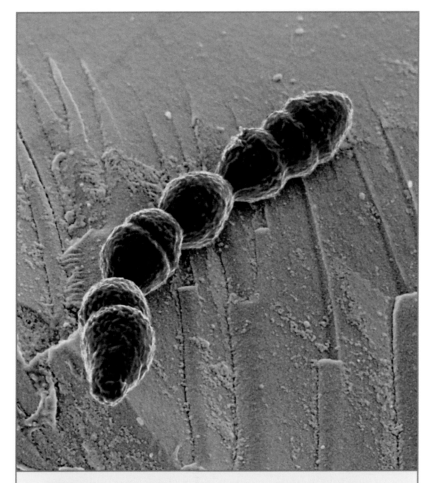

Figure 3.4 Meningitis can be caused by a bacterium called *Streptococcus pneumoniae.* This type of bacteria is routinely found living on the skin and mucous membranes. If the bacteria breach the body's defenses, they can cause meningitis. This micrograph of *Streptococcus pneumoniae* shows the bacterium's "twisted chain" structure.

people domesticated animals, or kept them in close quarters such as barns, kennels, pastures, and pens. They also believe that the diseases became more common when humans domesticated the animals. It is thought that people then

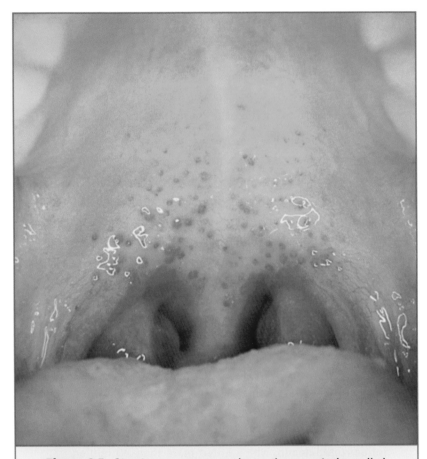

Figure 3.5 *Streptococcus pneumoniae* produces exotoxins called pyrogens, which can cause fever and rash. This is the throat of a person with strep throat, which is also caused by the bacterium. The red rash is easy to see here.

picked up the bacteria through continuous contact with the live animals or by handling food made from the animals. The bacteria then proceeded to cause similar or new diseases in people.

As mentioned above, only certain types of *Haemophilus influenzae, Neisseria meningitidis,* and *Streptococcus pneumoniae* cause meningitis. These different types came about from mutations that changed certain characteristics of the bacteria. For example, the mutation that formed Hib changed the surface of the bacterium. This change made the bacterium better able to attack the meninges. There are many mutations found in *Streptococcus* that alter the characteristics of their secretions. Some of these mutations cause them to

EMERGING DISEASES

Although disease outbreaks are more and more becoming a common fact of life, they are certainly nothing new. Ancient documents mention scourges that plagued people with a variety of ailments. Black plague, cholera, flu, measles, and tuberculosis have all appeared at particular times in human history. Scientists believe the lack of records of these diseases before a certain era indicates that the diseases did not exist in humans before that time. They have found evidence, however, that the emergence of these diseases in humans resulted from contact with domesticated animals. For example, influenza did not plague people until the domestication of pigs, which naturally carry flu. It is known that the 1918–1919 influenza epidemic, which killed more than 20 million people worldwide, originated from pigs. Dogs are believed to have passed along to humans a severe childhood respiratory disease called pertussis (or whooping cough). Measles are believed to have spread from cattle to humans when the first cows were raised for meat and milk by ancient civilizations in the Middle East. In more recent times, the HIV virus, which can lead to AIDS, is believed to have come from chimpanzees in Africa.

Many animals suffer from meningitis. The different types of meningitis that infect humans probably came produce secretions that protect them from the immune system's defenses. Other mutations create new secretions that permit the bacteria to invade the body more readily. These mutations, as we will see, also make the bacteria increasingly resistant to antibiotics and, thus, make the diseases they cause much more difficult to treat.

from several types of animals. Cattle, chickens, dogs, and horses most likely passed along their meningitis diseases to humans. The diseases spread to humans either by direct contact with the animals or through the bites of insects that feast on animal blood. Today, new diseases that cause outbreaks in humans are called **emerging diseases**. Some examples are Lyme disease, Legionnaires' disease, Hantavirus, and AIDS. Lyme disease is a bacterial illness acquired from the bite of ticks that feed on deer; Legionnaires' disease develops from air-conditioning systems that harbor soil bacteria; and Hantavirus spreads to humans from rodents. Scientists and health organizations that look for cures and treatments intensively study these diseases and how they are transmitted. For college students today, bacterial meningitis is an emerging disease. It is six times more likely to affect college students than other people. Scientists believe that the close conditions of classrooms, dormitories, and cafeterias make college students more likely to spread the disease. Plus, the high stress levels that college students endure weaken their immune systems, so they have trouble combating the microorganisms that cause meningitis.

4
Viral Meningitis

He did nothing in particular, and did it very well.
—Sir W. S. Gilbert, English playwright, 1836–1911

Viruses were not known during Sir W. S. Gilbert's time. However, his comment above adequately describes the life of a virus. Outside of a living host, viruses are nothing more than a simple container of **genetic material**, the chemicals responsible for heredity or the passing on of traits from organisms to their offspring. Unlike other microorganisms, viruses do not carry out any activities that indicate they are alive. Yet, once inside a host, viruses do a wonderful job of being alive by reproducing uncontrollably. They do this with little effort, using only the host's own resources. All viruses survive by living in the cells of other organisms. Viruses invade every type of organism, from the simplest bacterium to complex animals like humans. They are probably the most numerous organisms in the world. A drop of what appears to be clean seawater can contain thousands of viruses ready and waiting to invade a host. The bite of an aphid can pass along to an unsuspecting plant over hundreds of thousands of viruses that circulate in the insect's blood.

The same community near Houston that we discussed in Chapter 1 had a new meningitis scare in June 2003. This time, the area was threatened by a type of meningitis caused by a little-known virus. It all started when a dead bird found in Kingwood, Texas, tested positive for West Nile virus. This virus is believed to have been introduced to the New York City area from Africa in 1999. The virus normally spreads a mild disease between birds. American birds that are not accustomed to the introduced virus can succumb to a fatal inflammation of the brain called encephalitis. Normally, the virus cannot spread from birds to other animals. However, in this situation, mosquitoes were spreading the West Nile virus from infected birds to other animals, including humans. Some animals and people who were bitten by mosquitoes that had been infected with the virus became ill. Usually, they developed a fever and illness similar to a cold or flu. In some cases, however, the disease progressed to encephalitis and meningitis that caused paralysis.

WHAT IS A VIRUS?

Unlike any other organism, viruses are described simply as particles capable of causing disease. They have no cell structure and do not carry out any of the chemical reactions found in other organisms. Viruses are so small that they cannot be seen with the traditional light microscope used to identify bacteria and fungi. Light microscopes magnify small objects, making them easier to see. Viruses, however, must be viewed with electron microscopes. Electron microscopes work by passing **electrons**, small particles that are part of an atom, through the object being viewed. The electrons then strike a special screen that produces a black-and-white image of the object. Scientists then photograph the image on the screen. A

VIROIDS: SIMPLER THAN VIRUSES

It is hard to believe that there are organisms simpler and smaller than viruses, but there are. They are called viroids. Viroids cause a variety of diseases in animals and plants. They do not have a **capsid** and are composed merely of a small piece of **RNA**. Many viroids attack the nervous system, causing diseases related to meningitis. Viroids are very difficult to study because their RNA blends in with the chemistry of the host cell. Farmers suffered for many years as their crop plants were destroyed by viroids that were spread by insects.

light microscope can usually magnify objects 1,200 times their size. Electron microscopes can reach magnifications in the tens of thousands.

All viruses must live in the cells of other organisms, since they do not have the complexity to carry out the chemical reactions needed to live independently. After all, most viruses are made up merely of genetic material surrounded by a protein covering called a capsid (Figure 4.1). The capsid of the largest virus is no more than 1/10,000th of a millimeter long. Each type of virus possesses a characteristically unique capsid that can be identified with the electron microscope. Much of the capsid's job is to protect the genetic material inside. The virus cannot reproduce without its genetic material. Proteins called antigens give the capsid another role. Antigens are chemicals that stimulate the host's immune response. However, for a virus, antigens permit the capsid to find an appropriate host to live inside and reproduce. Antigens stick the virus to the surface of a host and help the virus enter the host cell, where it is able to reproduce.

Antigens on the capsid determine where a virus is going to affect the body. For example, cold viruses usually affect only the upper parts of the respiratory system because they specifically attach to cells lining the nose and throat. They cannot cause illness in other body cells, including the cells of the lungs. Likewise, the virus that causes hepatitis, a disease that inflames the liver, selectively attaches to liver cells. Viruses like West Nile virus can attach to a variety of cells and can live in different types of organisms. This makes them particularly dangerous because they spread rapidly by moving from one animal to another. Getting rid of the disease in one animal does not kill off the virus, because it can reside safely in the body of other animals that are not being treated for the disease.

Inside the capsid is the virus's genetic material. The genetic material of almost all organisms is composed of a chemical called deoxyribonucleic acid, or DNA. Many viruses use DNA

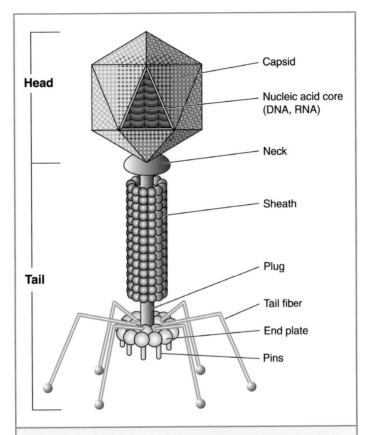

Figure 4.1 Viruses are organisms made up of DNA, a protein coat, and little else. They do not have the machinery necessary to reproduce on their own, so they must use a host cell. A type of virus called a bacteriophage is illustrated here.

as their genetic material. They are called **DNA viruses**. Other viruses lack DNA. They replace DNA with a related chemical called ribonucleic acid, or RNA. As might be expected, these are called **RNA viruses**. RNA is a more delicate chemical than DNA and is very likely to be destroyed by sunlight and common cleaning agents. Even sweat can destroy the RNA in viruses. This is not the case for most DNA viruses, which are more difficult to destroy.

Some DNA and RNA viruses are covered with a fatty covering called an envelope. Enveloped viruses enclose themselves in the outermost covering of the host cell, called the **cell membrane**. Thus, the envelope is not part of the virus but rather belongs to the host cell. The HIV and flu viruses are examples of enveloped viruses. The envelope helps them enter the host cell and provides better protection against the host's immune system.

Viruses reproduce differently from other organisms. They rely on the host to make multiple copies of their capsid and genetic material. Viruses begin reproduction once they enter a host cell. Inside the host, the virus's genetic material takes over some components of the host cell. The virus uses these components to build copies of its capsid and genetic material. Amazingly, the viral parts automatically come together to produce many new copies of the virus. This process, called self-assembly, starts when the proteins that make up the capsid create a case around the newly formed viral genetic material. Sometimes, the capsid takes up only bits and pieces of the viral genetic material, producing abnormal viruses. In some viruses, the viral genetic material takes up pieces of the host's DNA. This creates new varieties of viruses that either lose their ability to invade another host or gain the ability to produce new diseases.

VIRUSES THAT INFECT THE NERVOUS SYSTEM

A virus has to meet two conditions for it to infect the nervous system. First, it must have direct access to the nervous system. Viruses do not move on their own and cannot produce secretions to help them invade the body. Thus, they must be transported to the nervous system through the blood (or cells) or by direct placement in a nerve. Getting into the blood means entering the body through a wound, bite, or contact with body fluids. Second, the virus must have the correct chemistry to be taken in by nervous system cells. This means that the neurons

PRIONS

Prions are the newest organisms associated with emerging diseases of agricultural animals and humans. They were once thought to be a simple type of virus. Now we know that they are a unique virus-type organism composed of only a single protein. The first disease attributed to prions was discovered in the 1950s by researchers investigating a condition in the Fore people of New Guinea, an island north of Australia. The disease that the Fore named "kuru" caused severe deterioration of the brain that was more extreme than seen in encephalitis. Though it progressed more slowly than bacterial and viral diseases did, it always led to death. What was most confusing about the disease was the doctors' inability to find an **infectious** agent. Scientists eventually learned that the disease was caused by an infectious organism spread by the Fore ritual of eating the brains of dead relatives. A similar disease called "scrapie" was noted in sheep. Several physicians discovered that a disease just like kuru could be contracted through brain surgery.

In 1982, physician Stanley Prusiner discovered that an organism unlike any other caused scrapie. He named the organism a prion. A prion is just a small piece of self-replicating protein. Surprisingly, prions appear to reproduce without genetic material—that is, without any nucleic acids like DNA or RNA. Prusiner's finding opened the door for other studies investigating prion diseases. Now scientists know that a host of diseases, including mad cow disease (bovine spongiform encephalopathy) and certain brain diseases in humans, are caused by prions. Prusiner even provided evidence that prions might be responsible for one type of Alzheimer's disease, a slowly progressing brain disorder that causes memory loss and an inability to control body functions.

or neuroglial cells are tricked into letting the virus come across the cell membrane. Viruses are so small that they can leak out of the blood vessels into the central nervous system through small breaches in the meninges. These gaps open avenues to the central nervous system during infections with other pathogens or through normal wear and tear on the body. HIV makes its way to the brain this way. Viruses such as herpes invade nerves through openings in the skin or mucous membranes. Once inside a nerve, the herpes virus travels directly to other nerves and up to the central nervous system.

Polio, or infantile paralysis, was at one time a common deadly viral infection of the nervous system. Outbreaks of the disease in America and Europe during the first half of the 20th century crippled and paralyzed thousands of people. The name "polio" is a shortened form of the term *poliomyelitis*. **Myelitis** refers to inflammation of the peripheral nerve tracts and the spinal cord. There are three types of polioviruses now found throughout the world. The three types have slight variations in the antigens on their capsids. These RNA viruses belong to a group called the **enteroviruses** (*entero* means "intestine") because they primarily invade the digestive system. Enteroviruses enter the body through the mouth and multiply in the mucous membranes of the digestive and respiratory systems. Thus, they can be spread through coughing, drinking, eating, sneezing, and touching. The virus only causes poliomyelitis if it enters the bloodstream and passes into the nerves. Polio usually attacks motor nerves, where it destroys the neurons that carry messages from the brain to various muscles. The resulting paralysis can make the muscles used for breathing stop working. Luckily, the creation of a polio vaccine by Dr. Jonas Salk in 1955 caused a worldwide decline in this debilitating disease.

The rabies virus is the most infamous and misunderstood of the nervous system viruses. An RNA virus in the rhabdovirus group causes the disease. It almost always spreads through the bite of an infected animal, although there is some evidence that the virus can be infectious if inhaled. Bats, cats, dogs, horses, raccoons, and skunks can all carry rabies. An animal infected with the rabies virus is said to be "rabid." Rabid animals are usually very ill because the virus randomly destroys neurons throughout the central nervous system. The rapid advance of the virus throughout the nervous system usually causes a quick decline in health, leading to death. Almost all cases of rabies in both animals and humans are fatal. The first symptoms are flu-like and include body aches and nausea. Fever, hallucinations, and irritability develop as encephalitis sets in. In many cases, the eyes become sensitive to sunlight and the mouth produces thick, foaming saliva. Physicians and veterinarians notice that many infected individuals develop a distaste for water called hydrophobia. Luckily, it is possible to vaccinate against rabies. The vaccine does not cure the disease, but it lowers the chances that the virus will cause serious illness and death.

Herpes viruses are a diverse group of DNA viruses that usually infect the skin and mucous membranes. Most herpes viruses cause infectious rashes and sores on the skin and mucous membranes of the mouth and reproductive tract. Chicken pox, cold sores, genital herpes, and mononucleosis are four diseases caused by herpes viruses. The herpes simplex virus (HSV) group usually stays in the skin and mucous membranes. However, chicken pox that is caused by the varicella-zoster type of herpes can invade the central nervous system. It rarely causes disease in the nervous system, but it can use the nerve cells as a place to hide from the immune system and remain undetected for years or even a lifetime. Aging, illness, and stress can reactivate varicella-zoster virus in the nervous system to cause a disease called shingles. The Epstein-Barr type of herpes virus causes infectious mononucleosis. It was named after the two scientists who discovered the virus. Infectious mononucleosis usually affects the blood and immune system. It spreads readily through contact with infected saliva; thus, it got the name "kissing disease." Epstein-Barr virus is also known to cause a type of cancer called Burkitt's lymphoma and there is evidence that it can invade cells of the central nervous system.

ENCEPHALITIS AND MENINGITIS VIRUSES

A growing number of viruses worldwide specifically attack brain cells and the meninges. Viruses that selectively kill brain cells cause the disease encephalitis, while those that attack the meninges cause meningitis. Many viruses, however, can invade both the brain and meninges, causing a severe condition called meningoencephalitis.

Viral encephalitis occurs infrequently as small outbreaks spread out across a large region. Infants sometimes develop encephalitis when they pick up genital herpes viruses from infected mothers. The virus can pass through the placenta, the structure in animals that carries nutrients from the mother to the developing fetus. But it is most likely contracted during childbirth as the infant picks up the virus from the reproductive tract's mucous membrane. Biting insects and ticks spread a condition called epidemic viral encephalitis. The disease is caused by a large and diverse group of RNA viruses called arboviruses. Some of the best known arboviruses include West Nile virus, equine encephalitis virus, LaCrosse encephalitis virus, and St. Louis encephalitis virus. They mostly cause encephalitis and other ailments, including meningitis, in domesticated and wild animals. The death rate from viral encephalitis varies greatly. The disease can be so mild that many people do not even know they have contracted the condition.

Viral meningitis specifically targets cells in the meninges. It is much more common than bacterial meningitis. Luckily, the viral disease is not nearly as dangerous as the bacterial form. Few people are debilitated or die from viral meningitis. Any of the encephalitis viruses can cause meningitis that later develops into encephalitis. Small RNA viruses that are part of the enterovirus group cause most viral meningitis cases. The enterovirus group includes strangely named viruses such as the coxsackie viruses, echoviruses, and picarnoviruses. Picarnoviruses cause over half the cases of viral meningitis. The once common childhood illness called mumps is an enterovirus from the paramyxovirus group. Enteroviruses are highly **contagious**—that is, they spread readily from one organism to another through contact with infected body fluids. Viral meningitis progresses quickly after the virus incubates for one to two weeks in the body. During the incubation period, the virus reproduces until it reaches what is called a **critical population**, which is the number of viruses needed to cause disease.

A rapidly rising fever, sore throat, and vomiting are the first signs of viral meningitis. The symptoms usually include mild to severe headaches, chest pains, and neck pains. Stiffness of the neck and a rash will also accompany viral meningitis. Unlike in bacterial meningitis, there is little evidence of disease in the cerebrospinal fluid. Inflammation of the meninges is typically less severe in viral meningitis, and the body is usually able to repair any injury to the meninges caused by a viral attack. Usually, a particular grouping of signs and symptoms tells the physician which type of virus is causing the meningitis. For example, coxsackie viruses are more likely to cause chest pains. Echoviruses frequently produce a rash. A mumps virus infection is distinguished by swollen salivary glands. Almost all types of viral meningitis caused by enteroviruses can be controlled with proper handwashing. Meningitis that is spread by insect bites is best prevented by avoiding exposure to biting insects.

5

Other Types
of Meningitis

Disease is the retribution of outraged nature.
—Hosea Ballou, American clergyman, 1771–1852

Almost all scientists would disagree with Hosea Ballou's statement about disease. Hosea's view reflects an old-fashioned opinion that nature punished people who tried to go against its principles. Nature is not intentionally cruel and shows no outrage. Disease is merely an outcome of various creatures' competition for food and resources. Lions do not hunt with ill intent in mind. The antelope that is being pursued by a lion harbors no anger or resentment toward the lion. Similarly, microorganisms do not purposely harm the host while feeding and reproducing in the host's body. They are simply trying to survive. Meningitis is the outcome of the body's inability to control invasive microorganisms.

Bacteria and viruses are the primary causes of severe infectious human diseases in North America and Europe. Much of the reason for this has to do with the climate, native animals, and degree of technological development. Climate plays a big role in the number and types of microorganisms that can survive in the environment. Cold weather limits the growth and spread of microorganisms. Every microorganism has a preferred temperature at which it survives best. However, most microorganisms that cause disease feed faster and reproduce more quickly in warmer temperatures. Temperatures below freezing kill many types of microorganisms, leaving few, if any, to carry on the next generation. Thus, nations with high temperatures throughout the year have a greater abundance of microorganisms surviving in soil and water. Of all microorganisms, bacteria are most likely to survive in colder climates. Many bacteria produce structures called **spores** that permit them to survive the drying effects of freezing. Viruses do well in any climate because they have no living processes that are affected by temperature.

The native animals in an area establish the types of pathogenic organisms that can be transmitted to humans. Humans are vertebrates, animals with backbones and brains surrounded by a skull. Vertebrates include humans (and other mammals), birds, reptiles, amphibians, and various types of fish. The digestive systems of all vertebrates are very similar. The mucous membranes and chemistry are almost identical. Thus, it is possible to exchange digestive system microorganisms between different vertebrates. For example, *Salmonella* bacteria, which are common in the intestinal tracts of fish, are very easily transmitted to humans, where they cause intestinal disease. Humans belong to a group of warm-blooded vertebrates called mammals. Examples of mammals are antelope, apes, cattle, cats, dogs, elephants, pigs, and whales. Mammals have so many features in common that they frequently transfer pathogens between each other. The ringworm fungus commonly found in children normally grows in the fur of wild and domesticated mammals. Birds also can pass respiratory diseases back and forth with mammals. Regions where humans have a great deal of contact with related animals share many diseases.

Technological development decreases the populations of some microorganisms while at the same time increasing the prevalence of others. Most of the world's diseases are spread through sewage. Diarrheal diseases transmitted by sewage kill more children in developing nations than any other condition. Sewage treatment is a major technological advancement that has dramatically decreased the spread of disease. Food processing and sanitation technologies have also greatly reduced the spread of infectious food poisoning. Tightly packed housing and poor sanitation was mainly responsible for the rapid spread of the Black Death (also known as bubonic plague) throughout Europe from about 1346 to 1350. Plague is a bacterial disease of rats that spreads to humans through the bite of the rat flea. Rats take advantage of the comfort and food provided by human housing. This proximity to humans makes it easy for the plague microorganism to infect humans.

At times, technology that has improved our lives has also been known to spread disease. For example, Legionnaires' disease (legionellosis) is a respiratory illness that can be spread through air-conditioning and building ventilation systems.

The previous two chapters looked at the most common forms of infectious meningitis. However, other infectious agents can also cause meningitis. Recent cases of meningitis have been identified with microorganisms called fungi and protozoa. Fungi feed mostly on decaying or dead material. Protozoa usually eat other microorganisms or feed on dead organisms. Although most fungi and protozoa are harmless, a few are able to enter the bloodstream and are pathogenic.

FUNGAL DISEASES OF THE NERVOUS SYSTEM

Fungi represent an assorted group of organisms noted for feeding on decaying material. They begin the rotting process by secreting digestive juices that break down dead animals and plants. Dead organisms and animal wastes will not readily decay without the digestive actions of fungi. The broken down chemicals left behind by fungi become food for bacteria and protozoa. Fungi are made of complex cells covered by a rigid cell wall made of a special protein called chitin. Most organisms find chitin difficult to digest. This protects the fungal cells from their own digestive enzymes as well as from the digestive processes of other organisms. Fungi produce the greatest variety of digestive enzymes of any group of

DIABETES AND MENINGITIS

Diabetes is not one type of disease. It is a group of diseases that prevent the body from controlling the levels of sugar in the blood. The classical diabetes known as far back as ancient Egypt is a disorder that affects a gland called the pancreas. Today, it is called type 1 diabetes, or insulin-dependent diabetes. People with this condition are unable to produce enough of a hormone called insulin, a protein secreted by special cells in the pancreas. Most physicians believe that a genetic disorder somehow knocks out the beta cells that produce insulin. However, there is some evidence that certain bacterial and viral infections can also cause the body to destroy the pancreas's beta cells.

Another form of diabetes is called type 2 diabetes, or non-insulin-dependent diabetes. It is caused by an inability to use insulin properly. Most scientists believe it results from being overweight or from eating diets high in sugar. Some women develop this type of diabetes during pregnancy. High levels of sugar in the blood cause a variety of problems for the body. Some long-term effects of diabetes include blood vessel damage, loss of vision, kidney damage, and nervous system decay.

Physicians accidentally discovered a rare type of fungal meningitis resulting from diabetes. It began when a diabetic patient was hospitalized for severe headaches that led to unconsciousness. An examination revealed a common bread mold fungus growing in the patient's nose. The fungus does not normally cause disease. However, in this situation, the fungus took advantage of the high levels of sugar in the patient's mucous membranes. The fungus thrived on the sugar and subsequently invaded the brain and irritated the meninges. Unfortunately, the condition could not be treated and the patient died from brain damage.

organisms. As a result, they can digest almost any material, including leather and plastic. Fungal enzymes are valuable in industry, especially in chemical and food manufacturing. But they also permit fungi to invade the human body, making all of them potentially pathogenic.

Most fungi are composed of long branched chains of rectangular cells (Figure 5.1). Scientists call these chains of fungal cells **hyphae** (singular is *hypha*). Clumps of hyphae form the white fuzzy body of the fungus, called a **mycelium**. A type of fungus called **yeast** is made up of single oval cells. Some yeast can fuse their cells together to form a hypha strand. Almost all fungi produce special cells called spores. Many fungi produce the spores on the specialized structures we know as mushrooms. Spores are dried cells that permit fungi to survive under extreme environmental conditions. The spores will withstand conditions that would kill the regular fungal cells. This characteristic of spores makes it difficult to thoroughly rid clothing, food, and medicine of fungi. Another function of spores is that they help fungi spread easily from one place to another. Spores are easily carried by the wind and also make their way from place to place by sticking to feathers, fur, and skin. Fungal spores will break open to form a new fungal mycelium. People with mold allergies are allergic to the fungal spores that get into the nose and throat.

All animals and plants are subject to fungal diseases. Fungi are common soil inhabitants, and farmers lose many of the seeds they plant to fungal diseases called rots and wilts. Fungi called mildews and smuts regularly destroy corn, wheat, and other grains. One wheat fungus called ergot produces a hallucinogenic chemical that can cause illness and death. Stored fruits, seeds, and vegetables must be protected from the digestive activities of hundreds of fungi found on the harvested foods. Refrigeration does little to protect the foods. Every day, many people peer into their refrigerators to find colorful fungi growing on their food. Most of the food fungi will not harm us, and some are even

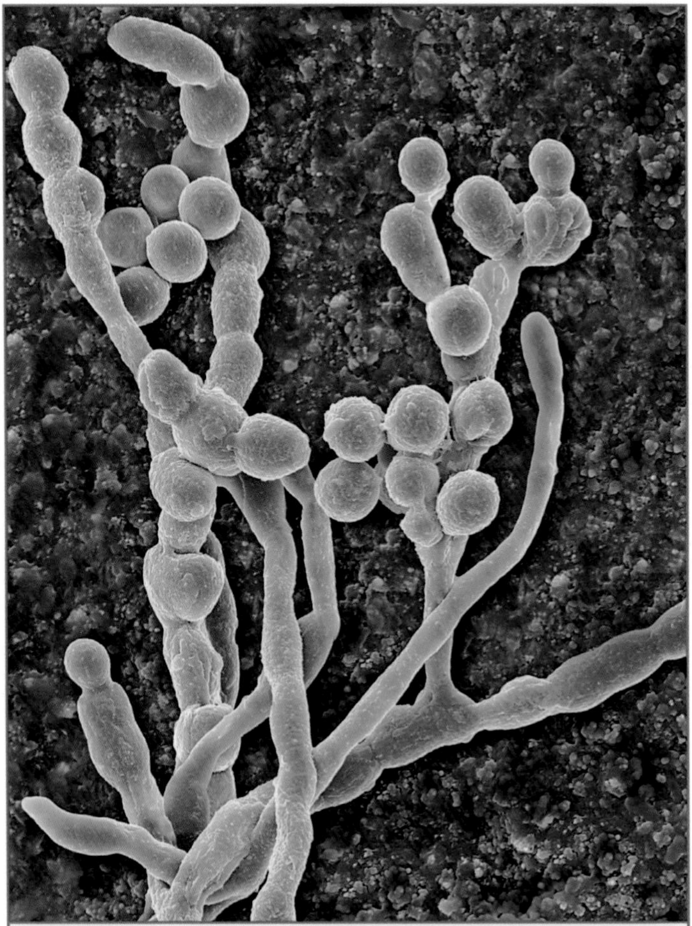

Figure 5.1 Fungi are composed of long strands of cells called hyphae. The hyphae form round spores, which can be seen at the end of the hyphae in this photograph. Fungi usually feed on decaying matter. Some will feed on body secretions, hair, and nails. These fungi have the ability to enter the body and cause disease.

edible and are used to flavor food. Cheese, soy sauce, and vinegar are made using the digestive activities of certain fungi.

Fungi have a more difficult time causing disease in animals than in plants. The immune systems of most animals are very effective at warding off fungal invasion. However, immune systems that have been weakened by other diseases or stress will permit fungal attack. The most benign fungal diseases of animals affect fur, hair, and skin. Fungi called dermatomycoses feed on the proteins found in skin and skin structures. The disease causes cats and dogs to lose patches of fur, and in humans it causes a mild skin irritation called ringworm (Figure 5.2). Many fungi are able to invade the respiratory system mucous membranes. Their lightweight spores are easily taken into the nose and mouth during breathing. These fungi can cause respiratory diseases if they make their way into the lungs. The digestive system and female reproductive tract in humans harbor naturally occurring fungi called *Candida albicans*, or candida yeast. This yeast usually causes few problems unless its growth gets out of control, in which case it can cause intestinal upset or irritation of the vagina, the lower portion of the female reproductive tract.

Fungi that get past the skin and mucous membranes can enter the bloodstream, setting the body up for meningitis. The yeast *Filobasidiella neoformans* (formerly called *Cryptococcus neoformans*) causes cryptococcal meningitis. Cryptococcus fungi commonly live in soil throughout the world. They are regularly found in the nasal passages of people who breathe in dust that contains infected soil. There is evidence that bird droppings also carry the fungi. This has led to strict regulations to reduce people's exposure to bird droppings. Special devices that discourage birds, in particular pigeons, from nesting and sitting can be found on bridges, buildings, and highway overpasses in many cities.

Cryptococcal meningitis begins when the fungi get into the blood by eroding the respiratory mucous membranes. The fungus does this through a variety of digestive enzymes that break down connections between the mucous membrane cells. Once it gets into the blood, the fungus causes fever, vomiting, and weight loss. The blood spreads the fungi to every body

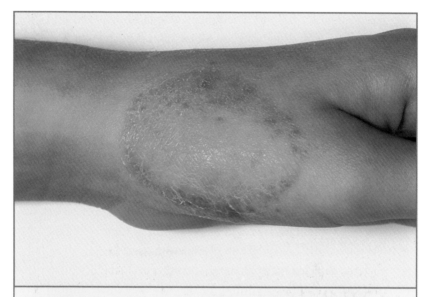

Figure 5.2 Fungi can cause a skin disease called ringworm, which shows up as a round, scaly patch of skin, as seen on this person's arm.

organ, where they cause severe damage. The initial signs and symptoms are followed by kidney and liver problems. Headache, paralysis, seizures, and possibly coma occur after fungal invasion of the meninges. Death usually results, even with treatment. Cryptococcal meningitis is not common in healthy people. Usually, it is people with AIDS and weakened immune systems who contract this condition. Half of all the cryptococcal meningitis cases reported in the United States are associated with AIDS patients.

Coccidiodes immitis is another fungus associated with fungal meningitis. It can live as yeast or as a mycelium. The yeast of the organism causes disease in animals. This soil fungus causes meningitis in the same fashion as *Filobasidiella neoformans.* Rare cases of encephalitis and meningitis have been attributed to fungi that normally cause respiratory disease. Histoplasmosis is a respiratory disease caused by the fungus

Histoplasma capsulatum. The fungus is found in bat and bird droppings. It is responsible for serious illness in children who touch or breathe in the droppings. The fungus will produce meningitis in severe conditions. *Candida albicans,* the yeast normally found in the intestines and the female reproductive tract, will also cause meningitis if it gets the opportunity to invade the blood. This fungus, however, rarely causes severe disease.

PROTOZOAN DISEASES OF THE NERVOUS SYSTEM

Protozoa are single-celled creatures that are abundant in soil and water. Some even live in extreme environments such as ice sheets, on mountaintops, and in the northern tundra regions. They are a very diverse group of organisms that feed on algae, bacteria, decaying material, fungi, and other protozoa. Scientists categorize protozoa according to the way they move around the environment. Only a small number of protozoa causes disease in humans. However, two of these diseases have major economic and health implications worldwide. Malaria and sleeping sickness are incurable protozoan conditions that cause more illness and economic loss than any other diseases. They commonly afflict people in Africa, Asia, Central America, the Middle East, South America, and Southern Europe. North America is home to two protozoan diseases—amoebic dysentery and giardiasis—that cause intestinal infections. The protozoa causing amoebic dysentery and giardiasis live in the intestines of many animals. People who drink water contaminated with animal droppings can contract these diseases.

Primary amoebic meningoencephalitis, or PAM, is a worldwide cause of encephalitis and meningitis. Two types of **amoebas**—shapeless protozoans that move around by crawling (Figure 5.3)—cause this disease. *Naegleria fowleri* is a common amoeba found in fresh water. The other protozoan that causes meningitis is *Acanthamoeba spp.* The "spp" means various species of this group. *Acanthamoeba* are usually associated with diseases of the eyes and skin. At one time,

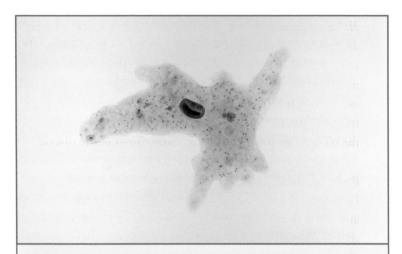

Figure 5.3 Amoebas are shapeless, single-celled organisms that can cause both encephalitis and meningitis. This is an amoeba, seen through a light microscope, magnified 36 times.

Acanthamoeba infections were caused by improperly maintained hot tubs. Several people developed the disease from hot tubs at health clubs and in homes. Both of these organisms cause a similar disease. The disease begins when the amoebas invade the nervous system through the blood. Sometimes, they enter the nervous system directly by passing through small openings in the upper part of the nose. These openings pass nerves that carry the sense of smell to the brain. Once inside the nervous system, the amoebas feed on and damage the brain cells and meninges. The disease almost always leads to death.

Naegleria fowleri is more infectious than *Acanthamoeba*. It has an amoeba form called a **trophozoite** that spends most of its time eating decaying material. *Naegleria* also has a swimming form called a swarmer. It swims using a whip-like structure called a **flagellum**. The swarmer can swim into the eyes, mouth, and nose, where it enters the body. It also produces a dormant form called a **cyst**. The cyst allows *Naegleria fowleri* to survive drying and attack by the body's immune defenses. Cysts will lodge in the mucous membranes and hatch out trophozoites that are ready to feed on living tissues. *Acanthamoeba* lives only as a trophozoite. However, it does produce a cyst that helps spread the amoeba from one body of water to another. *Acanthamoeba* cysts are easily carried on the feet. People who go into the water without washing soil or pond mud from their feet contaminate many pools with *Acanthamoeba*. The cysts of both *Acanthamoeba* and *Naegleria fowleri* allow them to survive in swimming pools until conditions are right to cause disease.

Another protozoan that invades the nervous system causes a disease known as sleeping sickness. Sleeping sickness is caused by several species of *Trypanosoma* found in Africa, Asia, and South America. The best-known form is African sleeping sickness. *Trypanosoma* causes mild blood diseases in many kinds of domesticated and wild animals. It is spread by the bite of blood-sucking insects, such as the tsetse fly. *Trypanosoma* uses its flagellum to swim around the blood, where it eats nutrients and creates toxic waste products. Much of the illness comes from the way the immune system attacks the invader. Toxic chemicals produced by white blood cells of the immune system cause the irritability and mental dullness associated with the disease. Some people feel so tired from the disease that they spend much of the time asleep; hence, the disease is called sleeping sickness. The illness can damage the meninges and can lead to encephalitis and meningitis.

UNUSUAL FORMS OF MENINGITIS

When most people think about worms, they think of earthworms. However, earthworms represent only a small portion of the worms found around the world. Flatworms and roundworms make up the majority of worms. They are found in almost every environment and many are highly specialized parasites. Trematodes and tapeworms are two groups of flatworms that cause disease. Most trematodes invade the body organs, getting around by burrowing throughout the body. Some are found

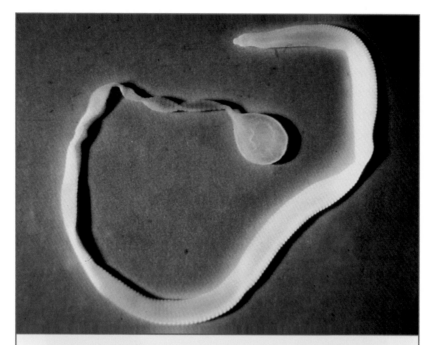

Figure 5.4 Certain types of worms, such as tapeworms (shown here) and roundworms, can cause disease in the central nervous system. Tapeworms themselves infect the intestines, not the brain or spinal cord, but they form cysts that can travel through the body and damage nerves and the brain.

in the blood, where they make their way to the liver and cause disease. A few trematodes damage the central nervous system by producing lesions in the meninges and brain. Tapeworms (Figure 5.4) are usually found in the intestine, where they eat any food they can take up. Most tapeworm infestations cause mild malnutrition. However, the cyst form of the tapeworm travels through the body, where it can lodge in various body parts. It is not unusual for tapeworm cysts to stray into the brain and nerves. The cyst can damage nerves as it grows, crushing neurons and neuroglial cells. There have been cases in which the cysts ended up in the brain and meninges, producing a form of encephalitis and meningitis.

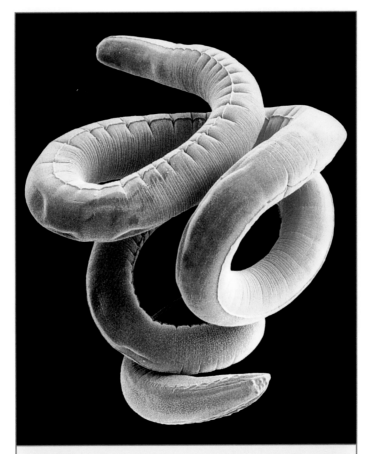

Figure 5.5 Roundworms can live in the blood of mammals, and can travel to the brain, where they can cause meningitis. This photograph of a roundworm, magnified 130 times, was taken with a scanning electron microscope.

Roundworms (Figure 5.5) are known to physicians, scientists, and veterinarians as **nematodes**. Most nematodes are microscopic worms that live in soil and water without causing disease. Many nematodes, however, invade the roots of plants, causing extensive damage to crops. A few nematodes cause disease in animals and humans. Most nematodes live in the digestive system, where they feed and reproduce. Others live in the blood and body organs, entering the body through insect bites and wounds. Parasitic nematodes are usually very small. However, a common nematode parasite of pigs called *Ascaris* can get as big as a pencil. *Ascaris* weaves its way through the body and can enter the meninges and the brain. It is not unusual to find people infected with *Ascaris*. In September 2000, the Centers for Disease Control (CDC) completed a study investigating a type of meningitis caused by *Baylisascaris procyonis*, a roundworm parasite found in raccoons. Several people in California, Illinois, Michigan, Minnesota, New York, Oregon, and Pennsylvania developed meningoencephalitis from *Baylisascaris procyonis*. It is believed the people picked up the nematode eggs from raccoon droppings. All of the cases occurred in cities where raccoons were living in buildings and nearby parks.

6

Epidemiology

As we advance in life, we learn the limits of our abilities.
—James A. Froude, English historian, 1818–1894

Epidemiology is defined as the study of disease transmission, a simple definition for a very difficult area of science. As scientists learn more about diseases, they also find out how difficult it is to keep diseases under control. The disease AIDS, for example, tests the limits of both our abilities and our knowledge. Volumes of books have been written about AIDS, and yet there is still no cure or vaccine, and the disease remains on the rise in Africa and Asia. The best understanding of the various types of meningitis still leaves outbreaks a mystery. Why did only certain children in the Houston area come down with bacterial meningitis? Why did the disease only take hold in certain schools? Why did meningitis not spread to others in the households of infected children? Why is it not possible to predict future outbreaks in the area? These questions plague many epidemiological investigations.

Any human disease that occurs throughout the world is studied by the Centers for Disease Control (CDC), located in in Atlanta, Georgia. The CDC is part of a larger U.S. government agency called the Department of Health and Human Services. Scientists and physicians perform many types of epidemiological research studies at the CDC facility. The CDC works together with the United Nations World Health Organization (WHO) to monitor the spread of disease. Both groups work with local public health organizations to prevent disease outbreaks and make recommendations about treatments. Vaccination programs developed by the CDC have nearly wiped out many childhood diseases that were once common throughout the United States. Few children today suffer from German measles, mumps, or whooping cough. The eradication of small-pox was one of the greatest challenges taken on by the CDC and WHO. Thanks to global vaccination programs, no new cases of smallpox have occurred since the 1970s. Currently, the WHO hopes to eliminate measles and polio over the next few years.

Epidemiologists are scientists who study epidemiology. Many epidemiologists do laboratory research to investigate the ways diseases occur. Others track the spread of disease using volumes of information collected from physicians, public health officials, and scientists. Epidemiologists use a precise set of terms to describe the spread of disease. They do this so they can steer clear of any confusion and misunderstanding of their findings. The meningitis cases in Houston caused a stir in the area because the media reported that an "outbreak" was occurring, even though what was happening did not fit the definition of *outbreak* used by epidemiologists. As a result, area public health officials were not at first willing to treat the incident as an outbreak. Public outcry caused the health agencies to assist with vaccination programs. People were upset that the agencies were not responding adequately. Yet, according to the CDC's definition of *outbreak,* the agencies were acting properly. Today, the CDC is quick to send out educational materials to ward off public panic and confusion.

THE VOCABULARY OF EPIDEMIOLOGY

Studying an infectious disease like meningitis requires an understanding of terms that precisely explain the spread of the disease. The first factor an epidemiologist must identify is whether or not the disease is communicable. **Communicable** means that the disease can be spread from one organism to another. Once scientists know the disease is communicable, they have to find the portals of entry and exit. **Portal of entry** refers to the area where the microorganism gets into the body to cause disease. Bacterial meningitis has one major portal of entry: It generally enters the blood through irritations in the mucous membranes. The portal of entry must be known to find ways to control the spread of the microorganism. The term **portal of exit** describes how the microorganism leaves the body to invade another host. Bacterial meningitis leaves the body through the mucus. This tells epidemiologists that the mucus of people who have meningitis is infectious and must be contained to reduce the spread of the disease. Viral meningitis has a different portal of exit from that of bacterial meningitis. It can only leave the body through blood taken up by a biting insect. This information tells public health agencies that they can reduce further spread of the disease by controlling populations of that particular biting insect.

Morbidity and *mortality* are two terms epidemiologists use when describing the severity of a disease. **Morbidity** means the number of people who become ill from a given disease. The morbidity of a disease is partially affected by the means of disease transmission. People exposed to biting insects, for example, have a greater risk of contracting viral meningitis. However, a person's age, gender, habits, health, past history of disease, and race influence morbidity. Bacterial meningitis usually has a low morbidity in a population of people (Figure 6.1). However, its morbidity in young people is greater than in the overall population. This tells epidemiologists that young people are more at risk for bacterial meningitis. The disease is also more prevalent and severe in people with weakened immune systems, and it spreads more quickly in underprivileged communities where many young people are malnourished.

Mortality refers to the rate of death from the disease. It can be reported as the percentage of people who die from the disease or as the number of people who die within a particular population. Mortality rates are determined for both treated and untreated people. This is particularly important when dealing with a disease such as meningitis, which is difficult to diagnose. Public health agencies know that they must work harder to obtain earlier diagnoses for diseases with high

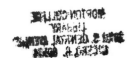

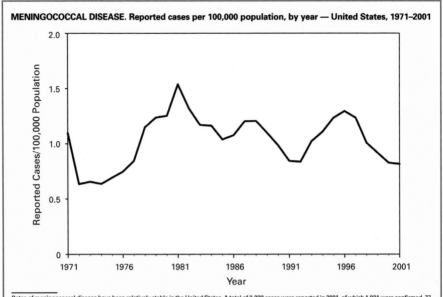

MENINGOCOCCAL DISEASE. Reported cases per 100,000 population, by year — United States, 1971–2001

Rates of meningococcal disease have been relatively stable in the United States. A total of 2,333 cases were reported in 2001, of which 1,931 were confirmed, 77 probable, seven suspected, and 318 of unknown case status. Serogroup information was reported for 33% of cases; serogroup Y accounted for 33% of those reported. Most other cases were caused by serogroup B (32%) or serogroup C (27%). Although rates of meningococcal disease are usually highest among children aged <1 year, 55% of cases in 2001 occurred among persons aged ≥18 years.

Figure 6.1 Between 1971 and 2001, morbidity rates—the number of people who get the disease—of meningitis were fairly low (rising to only about 1.5 cases per 100,000 people, or 0.0015%).

untreated mortalities. It is one goal of both the CDC and the WHO to reduce the mortality of communicable and noncommunicable diseases. One way to do this is to prevent the spread of the disease. For example, comprehensive AIDS awareness programs developed by these agencies have been carried out worldwide to reduce the transmission of AIDS. Another way to reduce mortality is through therapeutic treatments. Development of new drugs has significantly reduced the suffering of people with AIDS. To be treated for a disease, however, it must first be recognized. Unfortunately, many people die from bacterial meningitis before it is reported and treated. Fortunately, common antibiotic drug treatments can reduce the disease's mortality once the case is identified as meningitis.

The epidemiology of the different types of meningitis involves other terms that help describe how they spread. **Attack rate** describes the number of people who get ill after exposure to the disease. This is not always a simple number to calculate. Bacterial meningitis spreads directly from one person to another. Thus, it is possible to figure out how many people were exposed to the infected individual. The bacterial meningitis infections in the Houston area affected schoolchildren. In this case, it was not difficult to collect the names of the children and family members who had been in contact with the affected individuals. Public health agencies were able to monitor the exposed people to thwart additional cases of meningitis. On the other hand, it is very difficult to calculate the attack rate for viral meningitis, which is spread by insect bites. Exposure to an infected individual does not qualify as exposure to the disease. In addition, if someone was exposed to biting insects, it does not necessarily mean that he or she was actually bitten or that the biting insect carried the viruses that cause meningitis. In order to know the attack rate, public health agencies would have to know how many people got ill out of *all* the people who were bitten by infected biting insects.

As mentioned earlier, the epidemiological term *outbreak* has a specific meaning. It is defined as a designated number of cases occurring in a certain region within a specific length of time. Common diseases such as the cold require large numbers of people in a small area to be affected before being considered an outbreak. More unusual diseases such as bacterial meningitis are considered outbreaks when a moderate number of people are afflicted. Bacterial meningitis is referred to as being at the outbreak level when at least 40 people in a community of 100,000 are affected. Scientists must be careful when measuring outbreak numbers. The type of person who contracts bacterial meningitis should be kept in mind. The disease is more prevalent in younger people. The outbreak rate should be measured in that population and not include people who will not likely contract the disease.

Outbreaks that occur at levels much higher than the expected rate are called **epidemics**. Epidemics prompt immediate attention from local public health agencies, the CDC, and the WHO. Unchecked epidemics can overrun hospitals with sick people and cause public panic. The large number of people in the Houston area seeking bacterial meningitis vaccinations produced a temporary shortage of vaccine in the region. Only certain centers received vaccine to ensure that only those people who had been exposed to the disease were vaccinated. Epidemics that travel across large areas or occur throughout the world within a particular period of time are called **pandemics**. Pandemics frighten governments because they indicate that a disease is spreading out of control. Smallpox was once a deadly pandemic disease that has been wiped out through the cooperation of many governments. Another term, **endemic**, refers to a disease that is always present to some extent in an area. The common cold is a endemic disease that appears regularly in many places. Cases of the cold are usually restricted to small areas where it spreads quickly and then seems to go away on its own.

A MULTITUDE OF DISEASES

As mentioned in the previous chapters, meningitis is not just one disease. It is caused by a variety of organisms, all of which have unique ways of spreading and producing illness. Thus, the epidemiology of each type of meningitis must be examined separately. This also makes it important for physicians to identify the type of condition or organism causing the meningitis. It would be useless to treat viral meningitis with the same precautions and treatments needed to treat bacterial meningitis. Unfortunately, for a disease such as meningitis, it might take two days to confirm the cause. The patient could easily die before the proper treatment is administered. To speed up the diagnosis of meningitis, physicians look at the epidemiology as a clue to the type of organism that is causing a particular case or outbreak.

In May 2003, the Meningitis Research Foundation of the United Kingdom used epidemiological information to broadcast a public warning. The foundation noted that travelers going to particular regions of the Middle East were at risk of endemic meningitis. Endemic meningitis frequently breaks out in local populations. The disease is present all the time and can be contracted by travelers to the region. The foundation put out an advisory in 18 different languages at a time when it knew Islamic citizens of the United Kingdom would be visiting Saudi Arabia for religious observances. The advisory recommended that people visiting any Middle Eastern country get a specific vaccination for the type of meningitis endemic in the region. The foundation also gave information about the warning signs and symptoms of the particular type of meningitis in question. Because of this action, meningitis from Saudi Arabia was not brought into the United Kingdom by returning travelers. This precaution on the part of the Meningitis Research Foundation averted a possible outbreak of a disease that the United Kingdom would have been hard-pressed to combat. However, the advisory in this situation was effective *only* because the agency knew the type of organism causing the meningitis.

BACTERIAL MENINGITIS

As discussed earlier, three types of bacteria are responsible for most cases of bacterial meningitis: *Haemophilus influenzae, Neisseria meningitidis,* and *Streptococcus pneumoniae. H. influenzae* is commonly found in the respiratory system of healthy animals and people, making it difficult for epidemiologists to determine its attack rate accurately. Meningitis from *H. influenzae* occurs so infrequently that the attack rate comes out to an insignificantly low number. The organism is more likely to cause pneumonia than meningitis. Little is known about how easily it spreads from one person to another, which makes it difficult to predict who will develop the disease next. Further complicating the matter is that the b form of

H. influenzae is known to cause about 50 meningitis cases per year in the United States. Only 2 to 15% of the population may carry a particular type of *H. influenzae* called Hib. Public health officials need a way to distinguish the Hib form from other types of *H. influenzae* in order to predict a person's chance of getting meningitis. Tests for detecting *H. influenzae* Hib are available. However, they are difficult and expensive to perform. The tests are only carried out in medical technology laboratories with the proper equipment and expertise. Because *H. influenzae* Hib is endemic throughout the world,

DEMONS AND DISEASE

People today take it for granted that microorganisms cause infectious diseases. It is also assumed that public health officials will take rational steps to prevent the spread of disease. However, before the advent of modern medicine, people believed infectious diseases were caused by evil spirits and sinful behavior. Clergy and shamans applied their knowledge of culture and religion to ward off diseases. A common practice in Europe during the Middle Ages was to frighten away disease using fire and noise. Young men ran through the forests and fields at night carrying lanterns and torches while making loud noises with cowbells, horns, and whips. Indigenous people living on many Pacific islands used boats to rid the community of disease. Everyone in the community shouted their ailments toward a boat that was then sent off to sea, intended to take all the diseases along with it. Related cultures placed objects representing disease into a large pot that was then poured into a river or the sea. In India and Southeast Asia, it was common to touch a coin or another valuable object. The people believed that the disease was then transferred to the item. People then placed the object in the road where another person would pick it up and carry away the disease.

it would be difficult to eradicate it from every person in every nation.

The prevalence of *H. influenzae* Hib worldwide made the disease a good candidate for controlling through vaccination. Today, children in many countries are vaccinated against the bacterium. In addition, public health agencies are quick to vaccinate vulnerable people when cases start to appear more frequently than usual in an area. Vaccination has greatly reduced the incidence of *H. influenzae* Hib. It is now rare to see many cases and outbreaks are highly unlikely.

There are 13 types of *Neisseria meningitidis*, each of which is called a serotype. **Serotype** refers to a form of testing used to identify unique proteins found on the surfaces of bacteria. Scientists learned that three serotypes of *Neisseria meningitidis* cause over 90% of the approximately 140 meningococcal meningitis cases that break out each year in the United States. *Neisseria meningitidis* is not as common in the body as *H. influenzae* is. The bacterium is found mostly in people who live in airtight homes or spend a lot of time in crowded rooms. Many homes in North America are made airtight to prevent air-conditioned or heated air from escaping. Knowing this makes it easier for epidemiologists to predict meningococcal meningitis outbreaks. They know that is especially likely to show up in colleges, dormitories, military barracks, and schools. The attack rate is also easy to predict because most people who acquire one of the three *Neisseria meningitidis* serotypes become ill. This bacterium's knack for causing disease classifies it as a pathogen.

Streptococcus pneumoniae, as its name implies, is a pathogen associated with pneumonia. The bacterium is also most common in airtight homes and crowded rooms. Unfortunately, it is also frequently spread throughout hospitals and medical clinics. Most hospitals today use special air-conditioning filters to capture *S. pneumoniae*. Adults are more likely to get bacterial meningitis from *Streptococcus pneumoniae* than from the other meningitis-causing bacteria. Infection with *S. pneumoniae*, however, rarely leads to meningitis. People are much more likely to suffer ailments of the ears, eyes, nose, lungs, and throat than they are to contract meningitis. It is easy for physicians to calculate an attack rate for some types of disease caused by *S. pneumoniae*. However, it is very difficult to predict whether the disease will lead to meningitis. As a result, physicians look at indicators such as the general health and age of the patient to forecast if the disease might progress to meningitis. *S. pneumoniae* is found worldwide and creates pockets of disease, particularly among malnourished and poor populations.

OTHER CAUSES OF MENINGITIS
Specific types of biting insects spread all of the viruses that cause viral meningitis. The epidemiology of the disease,

ANTIBIOTIC RESISTANCE

In the 1960s, physicians treated childhood ear infections as if bacteria caused them all. There was no simple way to check whether the cause of the ear infection was a bacterium, virus, or some other microorganism. To make the process easier, physicians treated virtually all infections with **antibiotics**, believing that even if the drugs did not help the child, they would not cause harm. However, their belief about the harmlessness of the antibiotics turned out to be dangerously incorrect. The overuse of antibiotics has led to the development of antibiotic-resistant bacteria.

Whenever antibiotics are used to kill a bacterial infection, not all of the bacteria actually die. The strongest survive, although not in sufficient numbers to keep causing illness. Over time, these strong bacteria develop traits that allow them to avoid being killed by antibiotics. As a result, it is now more difficult, if not impossible, to treat certain bacterial diseases.

therefore, depends on the environmental conditions needed for the insects to survive. Mosquitoes need water to breed. Their young live underwater, feeding on microorganisms. Areas where mosquitoes are known to spread meningitis usually have regulations that control mosquito populations. Many cities in Alabama, Louisiana, Mississippi, and Texas spray swampy areas with pesticides to kill young mosquitoes. There are also regulations that prevent people from having too much standing water around their businesses and homes. The Texas Senate recently passed a bill that requires businesses to eliminate any conditions that allow mosquitoes to breed— there must be no standing water on buildings, drains, equipment, and loading docks. Texas was eager to pass this legislation because of the rise in the types of viral meningitis spread by mosquitoes. Biting flies and other insects that spread viral meningitis are more difficult to control. There is no single place to spray pesticide to kill these kinds of insects. Plus, their breeding would be difficult to stop because it is not limited to a single environment, such as a body of water. The best control epidemiologists can recommend today is to educate people about the insects and how to avoid them.

Fungi cause the rarest form of meningitis. In addition, they are very difficult to control and treat. Epidemiologists have a hard time defining the attack rate and morbidity of fungal diseases because information about them is scarce. There are not enough outbreaks to provide the data needed to make comprehensive calculations and predictions about the spread of the disease. Scientists do know that meningitis caused by the fungus *Filobasidiella neoformans* is mainly associated with bird droppings. However, they do not know if limiting exposure to bird droppings diminishes the disease. After all, the fungus is naturally found in soil and is known to travel long distances in the wind. Fungal respiratory diseases are linked to dust storms. However, the likelihood that meningitis will occur from this type of infection is unknown. This holds true for the other fungi as well, except *Candida albicans*, which is a natural inhabitant of the body. Everybody carries this organism with little chance that it will cause meningitis. The epidemiology of meningitis caused by candida yeast is based on health and gender differences. People with weakened immune systems are likely to have the fungus invade the blood and meninges. Females have a larger population of *Candida albicans* in their bodies than males do. Plus, it is carried in the vaginal tract where the fungus can gain easy access to the blood if the area is irritated or injured.

The epidemiology of meningitis due to protozoa and worm infections is highly specific to the particular organisms that cause the meningitis. Trypanosomes are usually found in tropical areas and are spread by biting insects. However, the organisms are commonly found in domesticated and wild animals, and cause few, if any, disease signs and symptoms. Thus, controlling the insects in tropical areas does not necessarily get rid of the organisms. Disease control is extremely difficult. First, it is not possible to kill off all the insects, and second, the organisms can reside in other animals until they can spread to the human population again. The WHO does have active pest control programs that reduce the numbers of insects living around humans. The organization also encourages the treatment of domesticated cattle.Travel warnings are put out to tell people to avoid areas with large infestations among the local wildlife. Insects are regularly monitored in these regions to check the spread of the protozoa and worms.

7

Diagnosis, Treatment, and Prevention

The nearer any disease approaches to a crisis, the nearer it is to a cure.
—Thomas Paine, American political writer, 1737–1809

Thomas Paine was right on target with his comment about society's motivations for paying attention to diseases. AIDS activists argued in the early 1990s that public health officials had not come up with serious treatments for the disease until the epidemic had reached staggering proportions. Warning labels were not placed on alcohol or cigarettes until their health effects reached alarming levels. Most types of meningitis can be prevented and have adequate treatments. However, people do not think about contracting meningitis until a series of cases erupts in their area. Few people near Houston were concerned about bacterial meningitis until the purported outbreak occurred. Even public health officials were caught off-guard. Many of the people in the high-risk group—school-age children—were never vaccinated. Vaccination recommendations were not strictly imposed because no cases were ever reported in the area. Thus, it did not seem necessary to enforce the vaccination of young adults until this time.

As discussed earlier, strategies for diagnosing, treating, and preventing diseases such as meningitis would not be possible without epidemiological research. Epidemiologists performing microbiology research study the life cycle of disease microorganisms. **Life cycle** refers to how an organism spends its life. Knowledge about the life cycle tells scientists about the conditions needed for the microorganism to survive. This information helps scientists prevent disease by finding ways to disrupt a microorganism's life cycle. How the microorganism spreads is an important part of the life cycle. Thus, interrupting the conditions it needs to spread can halt the transmission of a disease. Further investigation into the microorganism's life cycle and genetic composition provides physicians with disease treatments. A typical treatment kills or slows down the replication of the microorganism. Some treatments change the microorganism in a manner that inhibits its spread. Drugs given for viruses normally block the virus from getting into cells where it reproduces. Bacteria, fungi, and protozoa are usually treated by killing them with drugs.

Epidemiology teaches physicians and scientists enough about a disease to come up with an accurate diagnosis, effective treatments, and a prevention strategy. Each of these activities, however, is complicated by the fact that there are so many and varied diseases and causes of meningitis.

DIAGNOSIS

Diagnosis refers to the identification of a disease. Physicians use past experiences with many diseases to come up with a diagnosis for each disease condition. A diagnosis can involve a simple examination of a patient's signs and symptoms. For example, a physician can look for a fever and rash to determine that the disease involves an allergen or a toxin. However, this information does not provide enough information to find the specific cause of many diseases. Meningitis fits into the category of diseases that cannot be identified solely on an examination. Almost all forms of meningitis begin with what appears to be a common cold or respiratory disease. The disease then progresses to a septic condition that can turn into meningitis. This progression is typical of the three bacteria that cause meningitis. Thus, in addition to a physical examination, clinical laboratory tests must be done to hone in on the specific diagnosis.

Meningitis is a difficult disease to identify at first. This abridged excerpt, written in 2001 for the Immunization Action Coalition by Carla Newby shows the problem with diagnosing the disease:

> My nightmare began on Monday, October 26. Jake [Carla's son] was feeling ill when I went in to wake him and his sister, Lacey, for school. I gave him some ibuprofen and he lay around for the rest of the day. About 5 P.M. he said he really didn't feel well. He had a fever. I bathed him with cool water and held him. When I discovered his temperature was 104.5, I called our family physician and told him that I wanted to take Jacob to the ER [emergency room]. The doctor discouraged me, but I finally convinced him. At the hospital, they took blood and confirmed there was an infection somewhere. More tests were ordered and came back negative. The ER doctor diagnosed Jacob with strep throat and gave us a very strong antibiotic. My mother was with us and asked the doctor check for meningitis or encephalitis. The doctor said she wasn't concerned about meningitis and that if Jacob wasn't better by Thursday, I should take him to our doctor. She thought Jacob would probably return to school on Thursday. . . . But, by 6 P.M. he [Jacob] said his head felt like it was going to crack open. He continued to get worse. . . . I talked to my doctor again and he told me to get Jacob to the ER right away. . . . [At the ER] I told the doctor I thought he had meningitis. She [the ER doctor] ordered a CAT scan and the results were normal. She finally decided to do a spinal tap—the only way to confirm meningitis. . . . Jacob was suffering from pneumococcal meningitis. . . . Fourteen hours later, two days after he first got sick, they pronounced Jacob brain dead. . . .

Jacob's diagnosis of meningitis came too late to save his life. Unfortunately, this is true for many cases of meningitis.

Each type of meningitis has its own diagnostic characteristics. Physicians must combine a thorough patient examination with the results of clinical testing to come up with a specific diagnosis. All types of meningitis are accompanied by a headache that quickly progresses from mild to severe. Also noticeable with meningitis is the feeling of a stiff neck (Figure 7.1). Patients usually complain of neck pain or are unable to move the neck. Both the headache and stiff neck occurring together alert physicians to meningitis. However, even these symptoms are not enough information to assume that the patient has meningitis.

Bacterial meningitis is usually indicated by any general illness that precedes the headache and stiff neck. The headache and stiff neck combination unfortunately means that the bacteria are already damaging the meninges and possibly the brain. Meningococcal meningitis from *Neisseria meningitidis* begins like a common cold. It starts out mild and then progresses to a fever with general body pain within one day to a week. A rash shows up on the skin of many people. *Haemophilus influenzae* usually produces a severe flu-like disease, accompanied by drowsiness and vomiting. It can progress to the fever, headache, and stiff neck stage within 12 hours. A sore throat and cold-like conditions are typical of pneumococcal meningitis from *Streptococcus pneumoniae*. It is likely to produce a rash and vomiting very quickly. Meningitis due to other bacteria may not produce the traditional meningitis symptoms. For example, *Listeria monocytogenes* begins like a digestive system disorder before leading to the headache and stiff neck.

The signs and symptoms of viral meningitis take from one to two weeks to manifest. It takes some time for the viruses to reach the numbers needed to produce disease. However, once in the blood, the viruses bring about a rapidly rising fever. With the fever comes the same type of headache and stiff neck found with bacterial meningitis. The headache and stiff

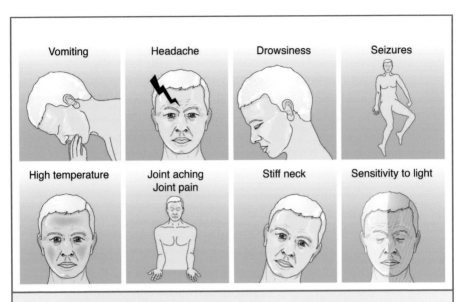

Figure 7.1 The symptoms of meningitis include nausea and vomiting, headache, fever, and stiff neck. It is important to see a doctor and get treatment immediately if meningitis is suspected.

neck tell the physician that the virus is attacking the meninges. Viral meningitis sometimes produces the cold-like symptoms, sore throat, and vomiting seen with bacterial meningitis. However, viral meningitis is not restricted to particular age groups, as bacterial meningitis is. Anyone exposed to animals, biting insects, and infected people that spread the diseases may be at risk. Physicians cannot always easily tell, however, if people were exposed to the disease through an animal bite. Insect bites are very difficult to find. Plus, many people do not remember if or when an insect bit them. Exposure to poliovirus meningitis is very rare. However, once detected, it is important to find the person who is spreading the disease. The disease is very infectious and will cause illness in unvaccinated people.

Meningitis caused by fungi, protozoa, and worms also produces headache and sniff neck symptoms. Though these symptoms are indistinguishable from the other types of meningitis, they usually follow noticeable damage to other body parts. These organisms will most likely cause disease or death before meningitis develops. Again, they are very difficult to diagnose from an examination in a physician's office or an emergency room. These diseases are very rare and occur in specific populations. Meningitis from protozoa and worms typically occurs in tropical nations. People who have traveled or lived in those areas are the most likely candidates to come down with these forms of meningitis. Some of the fungi that cause meningitis occur mainly in areas where people are exposed to the contaminated dust of bird droppings. Again, the physician must know the circumstances leading up the condition in order to make a judgment. Meningitis due to *Candida albicans* is more likely in females and in people with weakened immune systems. Otherwise, there is no other way of telling that this yeast is causing the disease.

Clinical tests usually start by taking a sample of the patient's blood and/or a culture of the infected tissue. There are dozens of chemicals that can be measured in blood. Physicians know that certain proportions of blood chemicals indicate either normal or diseased conditions. Sometimes, the presence of particular chemicals such as antibodies or antigens indicates an explicit disease. Different amounts of certain white blood cells can help further identify the cause of a disease.

Blood tests are given if the physician suspects that an illness is caused by microorganisms. Unfortunately, as in the case of Jacob Newby, blood tests are usually not performed unless the patient is showing serious symptoms. A standard blood test for infectious disease looks for a blood cell profile that indicates infection. Usually, an overall increase in white blood cells means there is an infection. This test is called a white blood cell differential test. Almost all septic infections cause an increase in white blood cells called neutrophils. These are the most common type of white blood cell and are the first to respond to infection. An increase in **monocytes**—white blood cells that help remove large particles from the blood and damaged tissues—usually indicates bacterial infection. However, some viruses, such as herpes, can also raise monocyte levels. Fungi, protozoa, and worms usually cause an increase in eosinophils. These cells produce secretions that help destroy large microorganisms. A host of diseases ranging from allergies to cancers can elevate white blood cell levels. This information must be combined with the examination to diagnose meningitis.

Special blood tests can determine if antibodies produced against particular microorganisms are present in the blood. Other tests can directly detect the microorganisms using chemical tests that identify specific antigens or toxins. However, these tests are time-consuming and expensive. In addition, they are not part of the normal battery of diagnostic tests for common diseases.

A **culture** involves collecting cells from the patient that may contain the infectious microorganism. The microorganisms are then grown or examined under special conditions that allow the physician to identify the disease agent. Bacteria and fungi are generally grown in culture plates and put through different tests that help scientists identity them. Skin tests can be performed to detect exposure to certain fungi such as those that cause coccidioidomycosis and histoplasmosis. However, these tests are not sensitive enough to confirm that the fungi are causing the meningitis. Viruses cannot be grown. They must be sent to special laboratories for testing. Protozoa and worms are large enough to be identified with microscopes. The specimens taken from the patient are compared to photographs with detailed descriptions of the organisms.

Cerebrospinal fluid analysis is the only test that can confirm the cause of meningitis. It indicates which microorganism is damaging the meninges. Blood tests indicate septicemia. However, they do not tell if the microorganism invading the blood is the same organism that is in the meninges. Cerebrospinal fluid analysis involves taking a sample of the fluid by injecting a needle into the meninges. A large needle is usually inserted between the lower back vertebral bones at a point where the meninges are exposed and unprotected by bone. The technique is called a lumbar puncture, also known as a spinal tap (Figure 7.2). The sample taken out is then placed into several sterile tubes that are analyzed in different tests. One tube is cultured to look for aerobibacteria known to cause meningitis. Another tube is cultured to selectively grow fungi. The third tube is used for Venereal Disease Research Laboratory (VDRL) testing. The VDRL test identifies the presence of sexually transmitted diseases. Another part of the sample is tested for the presence of viruses. Finally, the sample goes through a comprehensive analysis that looks for blood cell components and chemical evidence of meninges damage.

Protein levels in the cerebrospinal fluid of people with infectious forms of meningitis are higher than in healthy people. Bacterial meningitis usually shows the highest protein levels. Many of these proteins are bacterial secretions and immune system chemicals produced by white blood cells. Others are blood proteins leaking into the damaged meninges. The level of glucose, a sugar commonly used by the body for energy, is typically lower than normal in people with infectious meningitis. Viral meningitis is the exception to this. All micro-organisms, except viruses, use glucose. Instead, viruses deplete glucose, making it less available to the central nervous system. White blood cells, called leukocytes, are not present or are found in very low numbers in healthy people. People with infectious meningitis have large numbers of these cells trying to fight the disease. Bacterial and viral meningitis are usually indicated with more of one group of white blood cells called polymorphonucleocytes. White blood cells called lymphocytes are abundant with fungal and viral meningitis.

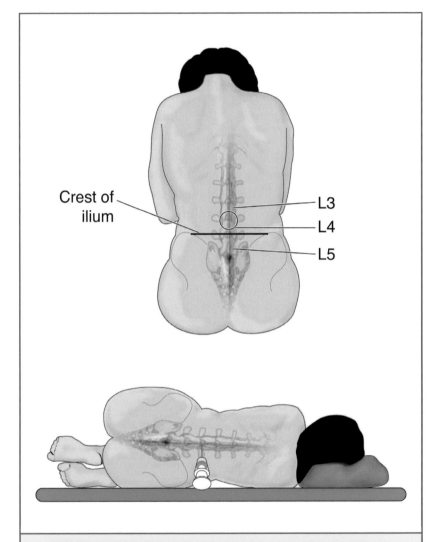

Crest of
ilium

L3
L4
L5

Figure 7.2 Taking a sample of cerebrospinal fluid for analysis is
the only definite way to tell if a person has meningitis. Normally,
cerebrospinal fluid is free of cells. The presence of red or white
blood cells, bacteria, or other particles such as proteins can
indicate severe disease. Doctors take a sample of cerebrospinal
fluid through a procedure called a lumbar puncture, or spinal tap.
A large needle is inserted at the base of the spine to collect the
fluid, as illustrated here.

Once a diagnosis of meningitis is confirmed, the physician is usually required to fill out a meningitis case investigation or reporting form. The form helps local public health agencies, the CDC, and the WHO track meningitis cases for epidemiological analysis. This tracking is called **surveillance**. A typical surveillance form asks for detailed information about the patient and includes a checklist of signs and symptoms. Also required is laboratory confirmation that identifies which organism is causing the meningitis. This process gathers the types of information needed for a more rapid diagnosis. It is also helpful for developing prevention programs.

TREATMENT

Meningitis is very difficult to treat. Part of the problem is that many of the drugs used to treat meningitis cannot cross the blood-brain barrier and, thus, have to be injected directly into the cerebrospinal fluid. Treatments can last from one to three weeks. The treatment is discontinued only when there is no chance that the microorganism will cause another infection. Even with adequate treatment, however, meningitis can lead to permanent brain damage or death. This is especially true if the patient enters a coma and shows extensive paralysis. To treat meningitis, doctors have to kill the microorganism and stabilize the body to reduce further damage to the meninges and other body organs. **Antimicrobial** chemicals such as antibiotics are sometimes given early in the diagnosis of illnesses that progress to meningitis. Most physicians prescribe antibiotics to kill off bacteria that may be causing the illness. Sometimes antibiotics are given to control bacteria that create problems during fungal and viral infections. However, these early antibiotic treatments do not always kill the microorganism that is causing the meningitis. Antibiotics are designed to kill only bacteria, and specific types of antibiotics will kill only particular types of bacteria. For example, the antibiotic ampicillin is most effective against gram-negative bacteria.

The antibiotic bacitracin is used in skin creams to control gram-positive bacteria.

Rifampin is the preferred antibiotic for treating people exposed to the different types of bacterial meningitis. It is not a cure, but rather an early treatment. The antibiotic is a preventive measure to keep meningitis from spreading between individuals. However, other antibiotics are given once disease is suspected. Ampicillin, cefotaxime, cephalosporin, chloramphenicol, deftriaxone, and gentamicin are given most commonly as an attempt to remove the bacteria from the body. Patients with severe meningitis are given large dosages of **intravenous** antibiotics—that is, the antibiotic is placed directly into the blood through a needle inserted in a vein. Unfortunately, some bacteria have developed resistance to all

HERBS AND HISTORY

Herbal medicine has been used in many cultures. Most anthropologists agree that people have used herbs to cure disease since before written history. The types of plants used in herbal medicine vary greatly between cultures. Many plants were selected as cures based on cultural beliefs. Herbal medicine in Europe was not always based on medical effectiveness. According to a principle called the "Doctrine of Signatures," the cure was believed to look like the ailment. Thus, a plant called liverwort was used as a remedy for liver disorders because the plant, which has lobes, looked like a liver. Plants with heart-shaped leaves were used to treat heart disease. Sometimes, pure metals such as mercury and gold were given to patients to purify the body. Much of the herbal medicine practiced in Europe did not work.

Most cultures, however, chose plants that they knew had medicinal properties. Many ancient herbal cures used in Asia and South America relied on plants containing chemicals that have since been incorporated into drugs used in modern medicine. For example, the aspirin used for headaches and the common antibiotics. Twenty years ago, penicillin was used to treat many bacterial diseases until the antibiotic became ineffective against certain bacteria. A powerful antibiotic called vancomycin was then used to kill these bacteria. Lately, some bacteria have developed vancomycin resistance. They must be treated with chemotherapy. Antibiotics are not trouble free. Many people develop allergic responses to mild antibiotics. Stronger antibiotics are known to cause kidney and liver damage.

Fungi are much more difficult to control than bacteria. They need to be treated with powerful **antifungals**, drugs that kill or slow the growth of fungi. Antimetabolites, azole drugs, and griseofulvin are some of the most common antifungal drugs. However, they can cause severe illness in the patient

other pains today is found in several plants that were used (typically chewed) to relieve pain. Tropical rain forests are home to many plants known to have value as medicines. New drugs for treating cancer and heart disease were taken from rain forest plants. These potential drug breakthroughs are one reason why it is very important to preserve what is left of the rain forests of Asia, Africa, Central America, and South America.

Today, herbal medicine remains popular among many people. Many of the plants used contain chemicals that supposedly cure various ailments. Meningitis has few useful herbal treatments, however. Most herbalists, or people who use herbal remedies, recommend black cohosh and scute for meningitis. Black cohosh is a root related to the buttercup and is given as a salve or powder. Scute is a type of mint. Pure silver, given as a liquid solution, is recommended along with the herbal treatment. It is important to be careful with this treatment, because there is no medical evidence that it actually helps cure meningitis.

and do not control large infections. Many pathogenic fungi become insensitive to the treatment when they form a growing pattern called a **biofilm**, which can somehow block the action of antimicrobial treatments. Fungi that cause meningitis form biofilms. Many antifungal treatments are experimental and are currently under investigation by an American governmental agency called the National Institutes of Health (NIH).

Protozoa and worms must also be treated with special drugs that are usually related to the chemotherapy agents used in cancer therapies. These treatments, called **antiparasitic chemotherapy**, involve drugs that can severely harm the patient. Antiviral drugs are available to control many types of viruses. However, these are very strong drugs that do not actually kill the virus but rather slow down its reproduction. They are no specific treatments for the viruses that cause meningitis.

Keeping the body stable is also a critical component of meningitis treatment. Physicians almost always provide over-the-counter or prescription drugs to reduce fever. Acetaminophen is the most common choice and it appears to be the safest drug to give to meningitis patients. It causes few side effects and does not interfere with antimicrobial treatments. Inflammation of the meninges and other body organs is controlled with anti-inflammatory drugs. Mild nonsteroidal anti-inflammatory drugs, called NSAIDs, are only used during the initial infection. Strong drugs called corticosteroids are used as the disease progresses. They may be given throughout the whole treatment until all signs of the disease have cleared up. Dexamethasone is most commonly used. Intravenous fluids to reduce dehydration are given to counteract vomiting. Sometimes nutrients are placed in the fluids if the patient has not been able to eat or keep food down. Other drugs may have to be given to control other signs and symptoms as they appear. Again, even the best treatment during the early stages of meningitis can sometimes leave a person blind, deaf, brain damaged, and/or paralyzed.

PREVENTION

Knowing the risk groups for meningitis is the first step in prevention. Each type of bacterial meningitis has a population of people who are susceptible to the disease. Newborn children rarely get meningitis from *H. influenzae, Neisseria meningitidis,* or *Streptococcus pneumoniae.* First, it is unusual for infants to encounter these organisms within the first few days of life. They are not common in the female reproductive tract or on the skin of the breast. Second, the mother's immune system passes along a temporary immunity to the infant while it is in the uterus. Most adult females are regularly exposed to *H. influenzae, Neisseria meningitidis,* and *Streptococcus pneumoniae.* Continuous contact with people throughout the day exposes adults to the bacteria. This provides a stronger immune response to the disease, thereby warding off a possible case of meningitis. However, infants become vulnerable to these bacteria once the maternal immunity wears off after a few weeks. In addition, exposure to the respiratory droplets of children and adults introduce bacteria into the infant's mucous membranes. Keeping a baby healthy decreases the chances of the infant's getting meningitis from this bacterial contact. A well-nourished and disease-free body helps the infant fight a septic infection.

Infants are more likely to get meningitis from bacteria that reside in the female reproductive tract and skin. The infants contract the meningitis bacteria as they pass through the vagina during birth. Meningitis from *Escherichia coli* and *Streptococcus agalactiae,* bacteria that inhabit these regions, can infect infants. Physicians have learned that women with large amounts of *E. coli* and *S. agalactiae* in the vagina have a high chance of giving birth to babies that develop meningitis. Knowing this, physicians can use prenatal care to prevent the occurrence of meningitis. Many physicians culture samples of the vagina's mucus toward the end of the pregnancy. Treatments are then given to women who have the *E. coli* and *S. agalactiae* bacteria. Such preventive methods are also used to control the spread of sexually transmitted diseases such as gonorrhea and syphilis. Unfortunately, not all prenatal diseases can be prevented with this type of strategy. Some disease microorganisms can pass to the baby through the mother's blood. This is true for many viral diseases, such as AIDS and German measles.

Vigilant vaccination programs that started in the 1980s reduced the incidence of *H. influenzae* type b meningitis in the United States. The disease was most prevalent in children until the advent of the program. By the mid-1990s, the disease had become associated with young adults and people over 60 years old. Public health officials in the Houston area suspected that *H. influenzae* type b was the culprit causing the meningitis cases in 2001, since it mostly affected high school students and elderly people. The few cases in young children occurred in unvaccinated families. The number of unvaccinated families in the Houston area startled public health agencies. Public health agencies and school officials had assumed that all children were getting vaccinated. Educational programs were promoted in areas where children were not vaccinated. A vaccine that was free to the public and inexpensive for the government was made available to poor families and people without health insurance. The vaccinations given to school-age children in the Houston area boosted the immune system. It helped make sure that the children's immune systems would effectively fight off even a severe *H. influenzae* type b infection.

Vaccines are drugs developed to strengthen the immune system's response to a particular microorganism. The Hib vaccine only works against a severe *H. influenzae* type b infection. Thus, the public health officials in the Houston area had to be sure that the severe *H. influenzae* type b was causing the meningitis cases. The vaccination program would have been useless if another bacterium was actually responsible. Hib vaccine stimulates the production of antibodies against proteins on the surface of *H. influenzae* type b. The antibodies stick to the bacterial surface, making it possible for the body to destroy and remove the bacterium. Vaccinations are not always effective against all *Neisseria meningitidis* and *Streptococcus pneumoniae*. However, new vaccines are effectively protecting young adults against all serotypes of *Neisseria meningitidis* except for serotype B. There are currently no vaccines available to prevent fungal, protozoan, and viral forms of meningitis. Personal hygiene programs are one strategy that reduces the need for vaccinations against types of meningitis spread by human contact. Many schools encourage children and young adults to wash their hands frequently to prevent the spread of infectious agents.

Prevention of fungal, protozoan, and viral meningitis is best done by controlling exposure to the animals that spread the microorganisms. Strict rabies vaccination laws ensure that the disease will not spread from pets to people. Mosquito control programs reduce the incidence of many forms of viral meningitis. Bird control in urban areas is also important because many birds carry fungi and viruses that can cause meningitis. Food handling laws make sure people who cook and serve food to the public do not spread viruses. Drug and food manufacturing facilities are regularly tested by government agencies to ensure that meningitis-causing organisms do not make their way into consumer products.

Meningitis can be a serious and even deadly disease that can strike without warning. However, as medical knowledge improves, it is becoming somewhat easier to diagnose, treat, and prevent this dangerous illness, which allows us to hope that someday meningitis will be, like smallpox and polio, a disease of the past.

Glossary

Amoeba—A type of protozoan that moves by crawling with structures called pseudopods.

Anthrax—A deadly disease of animals and humans caused by the bacterium *Bacillus anthracis.*

Antibiotics—Drugs capable of killing bacteria.

Antibody—A chemical produced by the immune system, used to fight disease.

Antifungal—A chemical or condition that kills or slows down the reproduction of fungi.

Antigen—A chemical that stimulates the immune system.

Antimicrobial—A chemical or condition that kills or slows down the reproduction of microorganisms.

Antiparasitic chemotherapy—The use of strong medicines to treat infections caused by protozoa and worms.

Arachnoid mater—The middle layer of the meninges.

Attack rate—An epidemiological term describing the number of people who become ill after exposure to the disease.

Autoimmune disease—A condition in which the body accidentally uses the immune system to attack itself.

Autonomic nervous system—A part of the peripheral nervous system that is under involuntary or unconscious control of the brain.

B cell—A lymphocyte that produces antibodies as part of the immune response to disease.

Biofilm—A film-like growth pattern produced by many bacteria and fungi.

Blood-brain barrier—A combination of blood vessels and nervous system cells that protect the brain from most harmful chemicals and microorganisms.

Brain—A part of the nervous system that controls body functions. It is located in the head and protected by the skull.

Brain stem—A section of the central nervous system located below the brain and just above the spinal cord.

Capsid—The protein covering surrounding the genetic material of viruses.

Cell membrane—A fatty covering surrounding a cell.

Central nervous system—Part of the nervous system composed of the brain and spinal cord.

Cerebellum—A small part of the brain located behind the cerebrum.

Cerebrospinal fluid—A protective secretion of the brain that lies between the central nervous system and the meninges.

Cerebrum—The largest section of the brain. The cerebrum controls movement and responses to senses.

Cocci—Spherical-shaped bacterial cells.

Communicable—Spread from one organism to another.

Conjunctivitis—An inflammation of the surface of the eye caused by *Haemophilus influenzae*.

Contagious—Readily spread from one organism to another.

Critical population—The number of organisms needed to have an effect on the body. Thousands of bacteria must be present in the blood before a person develops bacterial meningitis.

Culture—The growing of microorganisms in a laboratory.

Cyst—A dormant form of a cell. Cysts are usually covered with protective coverings.

Deoxyribonucleic acid (DNA)—The chemical that makes up the genetic material of most organisms.

Diagnosis—A medical term describing the identification and naming of a disease.

DNA—See **Deoxyribonucleic acid**.

DNA virus—A virus that uses DNA as its genetic material.

Dura mater—The outermost layer of the meninges.

Electrons—Small particles composing part of an atom.

Glossary

Emerging diseases—New diseases that are becoming prevalent in humans. They may be diseases transferred from animals to humans or new varieties of older diseases.

Encephalitis—Inflammation of the brain.

Endemic—Commonly present in a specific location.

Endotoxins—Poisons found in the cell wall of gram-negative bacteria.

Enterovirus—A virus that attacks the digestive system.

Enzyme—Protein that carries out certain functions for an organism, such as the chemical reactions needed for digestion and metabolism.

Eosinophil—A white blood cell that makes up part of the immune response. Eosinophils produce secretions that kill large invading microorganisms.

Epidemic—A disease outbreak that occurs in a larger than expected number of people.

Epidemiologist—A scientist who studies epidemiology.

Epidemiology—The study of the transmission of diseases.

Exotoxins—Bacterial secretions that cause disease in host organisms of pathogen bacteria.

Fever—An unusual rise in body temperature resulting from disease.

Flagellum—A whip-like structure on some cells used for swimming.

Genetic material—The chemicals in an organism responsible for heredity or the passing on of traits.

Gram stain—A laboratory technique used to indentify bacteria. It involves adding stains to bacteria to produce different colors based on the chemistry of the bacterium's outer covering. Gram-negative bacteria appear pink or red, while gram-positive bacteria appear purple under a microscope.

Hemolysins—Microbial enzymes that cause hemolysis, or the breakdown of red blood cells.

Hib—An abbreviation for *Haemophilus influenzae* type b, which can cause meningitis.

Host organism—An organism that serves as a place for other organisms to feed and live.

Hyphae—Chains of fungal cells. The singular form of the word is *hypha*.

Immune system—A complex system of body organs and cells that help recognize and fight off disease.

Infection—Invasion of the body by a disease organism.

Infectious—Able to spread throughout the body and travel from one organism to another.

Inflammation—A reaction to injury involving pain, reddening, and swelling.

Interferon—A chemical produced by the immune system that combats infections. Interferon is especially effective against viruses.

Intravenous—Placed into the blood through a needle inserted in a vein.

Life cycle—The way an organism lives from one generation to the next.

Lymphocyte—A group of white blood cells that defend against microorganisms that enter the body.

Macrophage—A white blood cell that destroys microorganisms in the body. Macrophages engulf the microorganism and stimulate the rest of the immune system.

Membrane—A covering surrounding a body structure.

Meninges—A protective covering, composed of three layers, that surrounds the central nervous system.

Meningitis—Inflammation of the meninges caused by disease.

Meningococcal meningitis—Meningitis caused by *Neisseria meningitidis.*

Meningoencephalitis—Inflammation of the meninges and the brain.

Microorganism—A small organism that can only be seen with a microscope. Algae, bacteria, molds, and protozoa are microorganisms.

Monocytes—Large white blood cells that make up the immune system. They remove foreign matter, including microorganisms, from the body.

Glossary

Morbidity—The number of people who become ill from a disease.

Mortality—The death rate from a disease.

Motor function—Body function that involves movement and the production of secretions.

Motor nerve—A nerve that controls and relays messages about movement.

Mucous membranes—Moist mucus-covered tissues lining the digestive, respiratory, reproductive, and urinary tracts.

Mucus—A thick, sticky fluid produced by mucous membranes.

Mycelium—Clump of hyphae that forms the body of a fungus.

Myelitis—Inflammation of the neuroglial cells covering the peripheral nerves and spinal cord.

Necrotic factors—Secretions in the blood that kill large microorganisms and diseased cells.

Nematode—Scientific name for a roundworm.

Nerve—A group of neurons and neuroglial cells that carry large amounts of information for the nervous system.

Nerve impulse—An electrical charge produced by a neuron.

Neuroglial cell—A nervous system cell that protects neurons and helps them function.

Neuron—Cells that carry out the jobs of the nervous system.

Neurotransmitters—Chemicals produced by neurons to send information from one neuron to another.

Neutrophil—An abundant white blood cell making up the immune system. It produces secretions that fight infection.

Outbreak—A nonmedical term referring to the sudden occurrence of many cases of a disease in a certain area.

Pandemic—An epidemic that occurs throughout the world.

Paralysis—The inability to move a muscle or groups of muscles.

Parasympathetic nervous system—A part of the autonomic nervous system that gets the body ready for action and slows down digestion.

Pathogen—An organism that causes disease in another organism.

Pathogenic—Able to cause disease in another organism.

Peripheral nervous system—The part of the nervous system that contains nerve cells that run throughout the body, outside of the central nervous system.

Pia mater—The innermost layer of the meninges, which directly covers the central nervous system.

Pinkeye—*See* **Conjunctivitis**.

Pneumonia—A respiratory system infection that causes inflammation and fluid buildup in the lungs.

Portal of entry—The area of the body where a microorganism enters to cause disease.

Portal of exit—The area of the body where the microorganism leaves to invade another host.

Prion—A virus-like organism composed only of a protein capable of replicating in cells.

Pyrogen—A fever-inducing chemical produced by the body or by microorganisms.

Reflex—An automatic response to something that stimulates the body.

Ribonucleic acid (RNA)—A complex chemical related to deoxyribonucleic acid (DNA).

RNA virus—A virus that uses RNA as its genetic material.

Saprotroph—An organism that feeds by digesting decaying material.

Schwann cell—A common neuroglial cell that helps neurons pass impulses.

Sebaceous glands—Oil-producing glands in the skin.

Glossary

Secretion—A substance produced by cells or microorganisms, made to flow out of the cell or organism.

Sensory nerve—A nerve found in the sensory nervous system.

Sensory receptor—A special nerve cell that interprets information from the environment.

Sensory structure—A part of the body that takes information from the environment and passes it along to neurons.

Serotype—A chemical difference caused by proteins covering the surface of an organism. Serotype is determined by laboratory tests that show how the serotype proteins interact with the human immune system.

Septicemia—The presence of microorganisms in the bloodstream.

Sign—A condition that can be measured or seen during diagnosis. Redness, sores, and swelling are examples of disease signs. Compare with **symptom**.

Somatic nervous system—A part of the peripheral nervous system that is under voluntary or conscious control of the brain.

Spinal cord—A portion of the central nervous system containing nerves that run from the brain down the length of the body.

Spore—A structure produced by microorganisms that helps them resist unfavorable environmental conditions. Under good conditions, spores develop into active microbial cells.

Surveillance—A term used to describe the tracking of the spread of a disease. Physicians are required to fill out surveillance forms that are then given to public health agencies so they can keep track of details about each case.

Sympathetic nervous system—A part of autonomic nervous system that puts the body at rest and aids digestion.

Symptom—A subjective condition that the patient reports. Dizziness, headache, nausea, and pain are examples of disease symptoms. Compare with **sign**.

T helper cell—A lymphocyte that stimulates the immune system to fight infection.

Trophozoite—A form of a protozoan cell that actively feeds.

Vaccine—A medication given to prevent a disease from infecting the body.

Yeast—A type of fungus composed of single oval-shaped cells.

Bibliography

Audesirk, T., G. Audesirk, and B.E. Byers. *Biology: Life on Earth,* 6th ed. Upper Saddle River, NJ: Prentice Hall, 2001.

Bauman, R. *Microbiology.* San Francisco: Pearson Education, 2002.

Brandileone, M.C., A.L. De Andrade, J.L. Di Fabio, M.L. Guerra, and R. Austrian. "Appropriateness of Pneumonococcal Conjugate Vaccine in Brazil: Potential Impact of Age and Clinical Diagnosis, with Emphasis on Meningitis." *Journal of Infectious Disease* 187(8) (2003): 1206–1212.

California Association for Medical Laboratory Technology Distance Learning Program. *Primary Amebic Meningoencephalitis (PAM).* Available online at *http://www.camlt.org/DL_web/930_PAM.html.*

Calvert, C. "Humble Students Get Vaccinations." *The Humble Observer.* (January 24, 2001), p. 1.

Daikos, G.L., T. Cleary, and M.A. Fischl. "Multidrug-Resistant Tuberculosis Meningitis in Patients with AIDS." *International Journal of Tuberculosis and Lung Disease* 7(4) (2003): 394–398.

Davies, P.A., and P.T. Rudd. *Neonatal Meningitis.* London: Cambridge University Press, 1995.

Gibbens, P. "West Nile Virus Now Confirmed in Kingwood." *The Kingwood Observer* (June 25, 2003), p. 1.

Kim, K.S. "Neurological Diseases: Pathogenesis of Bacterial Meningitis: From Bacteraemia to Neuronal Injury." *National Review of Neuroscience* 4(5) (2003): 376–385.

McVernon, J., P.D. Johnson, A.J. Pollard, M.P. Slack, and E.R. Moxon. "Immunologic Memory in Haemophilus influenzae Type b Conjugate Vaccine Failure." *Archives of Diseases in Childhood* 88(5) (2003): 379–383.

Nester, E.W., D.G. Anderson, C.E. Roberts, N.N. Pearsall, and M.T. Nester. *Microbiology: A Human Perspective.* New York: McGraw-Hill, 2001.

Newby, C. "Boy Dies of Pneumococcal Meningitis." Immunization Action Coalition. Available online at *http://www.immunize.org/stories/story40.htm.*

Parker, J.N., and P.M. Parker, eds. *The Official Patient's Sourcebook on Meningitis: A Revised and Updated Directory for the Internet Age.* San Diego: Icon Health Publishers, 2002.

Pollard, A.J., M.C.J. Maiden, and M. Levin, eds. *Meningococcal Disease: Methods and Protocols.* Totowa, NJ: Humana Press, 2001.

Samra, Z., H. Shmuely, E. Nahum, D. Paghis, and J. Den-Ari. "Use of NOW *Streptococcus pneumoniae* Urinary Antigen Test in Cerebrospinal Fluid for Rapid Diagnosis of Pneumonococcal Meningitis." *Diagnostic Microbiology and Infectious Disease* 45(4) (2003): 237–240.

Seeley, R.R., T.D. Stephens, and P. Tate. *Essentials of Anatomy and Physiology*, 3rd ed. New York: McGraw-Hill, 1999.

Verhaegen, J., S.J. Vandecasteele, J. Vandeven, N. Verbiest, K. Lagrou, and W.E. Peetermans. "Antibiotic Susceptibility and Serotype Distribution of 240 *Streptococcus pneumoniae* Causing Meningitis in Belgium, 1997–2000." *Acta Clinica Belgium* 58(1) (2003): 19–26.

Willett, E. *Meningitis*. Berkeley Heights, NJ: Enslow Publishers, Inc., 1999.

Wilson, H., O. Mansoor, J. Wenger, R. Martin, I. Zanardi, M. O'Leary, and V. Rabukawaqu. "Estimating the *Haemophilus influenzae* Type b (Hib) Disease Burden and the Impact of Hib Vaccine in Fiji." *Vaccine* 16; 21(17–18) (2003): 1907–1912.

Wood, S. "County Conducts Mass Vaccinations at HHS." *The Kingwood Observer* (January 31, 2001), p. 1.

World Health Organization. *Cerebrospinal Meningitis Control: Report*. New York: United Nations World Health Organization, 1976.

Further Reading

Bauman, R. *Microbiology*. San Francisco: Pearson Education, 2002.

Parker, J.N., and P.M. Parker, eds. *The Official Patient's Sourcebook on Meningitis: A Revised and Updated Directory for the Internet Age*. San Diego: Icon Health Publishers, 2002.

Roos, K.L. *Meningitis: 100 Maxims*. London: Edward Arnold Press, 1996.

Willett, E. *Meningitis*. Berkeley Heights, NJ: Enslow Publishers, Inc., 1999.

Centers for Disease Control
http://www.cdc.gov
Search "meningitis"

HealthLink. Medical College of Wisconsin
http://healthlink.mcw.edu
Search "meningitis"

Martin Memorial Health System
http://www.mmhs.com
Go to Health Library A–Z and search "meningitis"

Mayo Clinic.com
http://www.mayoclinic.com/invoke.cfm?id=DS00118

Medline Plus. A Service of the U.S. National Library of
Medicine and the National Institutes of Health
http://www.nlm.nih.gov/medlineplus/meningitis.html

Meningitis Foundation of America
http://www.musa.org

Meningitis Research Foundation
http://www.meningitis.org

Meningitis Trust
http://www.meningitis-schools.org.uk/index.html

National Foundation for Infectious Diseases
http://www.nfid.org/library/meningococcal

Public Broadcasting Service. Website for the *Nova* television
special "Killer Disease on Campus"
http://www.pbs.org/wgbh/nova/meningitis/resources.html
http://www.pbs.org/wgbh/nova/meningitis

World Health Organization
http://www.who.int/health-topics/meningitis.htm

Index

Index

Picture Credits

18: Lambda Science Artwork
19: Lambda Science Artwork
21: Lambda Science Artwork
26: Lambda Science Artwork
29: Lambda Science Artwork
35: Lambda Science Artwork
39: © Dr. Dennis Kunkel/Visuals Unlimited
41: © Dr. Dennis Kunkel/Visuals Unlimited
44: © Gary Gaugler/Visuals Unlimited
45: Courtesy Public Health Image Library (PHIL), CDC

51: Lambda Science Artwork
63: © Dr. Dennis Kunkel/Visuals Unlimited
65: © Mediscan/Visuals Unlimited
67: © Carolina Biological/Visuals Unlimited
69: © Larry Jensen/Visuals Unlimited
70: © Dr. Richard Kessel & Dr. Gene Shih /Visuals Unlimited
75: Courtesy *MMWR*, Vol. 50. No. 53, CDC
88: Lambda Science Artwork
92: Lambda Science Artwork

Cover: © Gary Gaugler/Visuals Unlimited

About the Author

Brian Shmaefsky is a professor of biology and environmental sciences at Kingwood College near Houston, Texas. He did his undergraduate studies in biology at Brooklyn in New York and completed masters and doctoral studies at Southern Illinois University at Edwardsville. His research emphasis is in environmental physiology. Dr. Shmaefsky has many publications on science education, some appearing in American Biology Teacher and the Journal of College Science Teaching. He regularly consults on general biology and microbiology textbook projects. Dr. Shmaefsky is also very active serving on environmental awareness and policy committees in Texas. He has two children Kathleen, 13, and Timothy, 15, and lives in Kingwood with his dog Dusty.

About the Editor

The late I. Edward Alcamo was a Distinguished Teaching Professor of Microbiology at the State University of New York at Farmingdale. Alcamo studied biology at Iona College in New York and earned his M.S. and Ph.D. degrees in microbiology at St. John's University, also in New York. He had taught at Farmingdale for over 30 years. In 2000, Alcamo won the Carski Award for Distinguished Teaching in Microbiology, the highest honor for microbiology teachers in the United States. He was a member of the American Society for Microbiology, the National Association of Biology Teachers, and the American Medical Writers Association. Alcamo authored numerous books on the subjects of microbiology, AIDS, and DNA technology as well as the award-winning textbook *Fundamentals of Microbiology*, now in its sixth edition.